D0959104

NATURAL HEALING REMEDIES

1999

NATURAL HEALING REMEDIES

The Smartest, Quickest Ways to Guard Your Health

Rodale Press, Inc.
Emmaus, Pennsylvania

Notice

This book is intended as a reference volume only, not as a medical manual. The information given here is designed to help you make informed decisions about your health. It is not intended as a substitute for any treatment that may have been prescribed by your doctor. If you suspect that you have a medical problem, we urge you to seek competent medical help.

Copyright © 1999 by Rodale Press, Inc.

Illustrations copyright © 1999 by Narda Lebo

All rights reserved. No part of this publication may be reproduced or transmitted in any form or by any means, electronic or mechanical, including photocopying, recording, or any other information storage and retrieval system, without the written permission of the publisher.

Printed in the United States of America on acid-free ∞ , recycled paper ♲

"Three Minutes to Total Relaxation" on page 82 was adapted from *The Three Minute Meditator* by David Harp and Nina Feldman, Ph.D. Copyright © 1996 by New Harbinger Publications. Reprinted with permission.

ISBN 1–57954–054–6 hardcover

Distributed to the book trade by St. Martin's Press

2   4   6   8   10   9   7   5   3   1   hardcover

─────── OUR PURPOSE ───────

"We inspire and enable people to improve their lives and the world around them."

Natural Healing Remedies 1999 Staff

Senior Managing Editor: Edward Claflin

Editor: Emrika Padus

Contributing Writers: Anne Alexander; Alisa Bauman; Colin Beavan; Kenneth Winston Caine; Rick Chillot; Erik D'Amato; Daryn Eller; Nina Feldman; Dorothy Foltz-Gray; Marisa Fox; Stephen C. George; Susan Flagg Godbey; Laura Goldstein; Greg Gutfeld; Toby Hanlon; David Harp; Joe Kita; Holly McCord; Mike McGrath; Michele Meyer; Peggy Morgan; Michele Morris; Miriam Nelson, Ph.D.; Cathy Perlmutter; Colleen Pierre, R.D.; Stephen Rae; Mark Remy; Sarah Robertson; Mark Roman; Maggie Spilner; Laurence Roy Stains; Michele Stanten; Nancy Stedman; Sharon Stocker; Varro E. Tyler, Ph.D., Sc.D.; Marion Winik; Yun Lee Wolfe; Selene Yeager

Associate Research Manager: Anita C. Small

Lead Researcher: Christine Dreisbach

Permissions Coordinator: Grete Haentjens

Senior Copy Editor: Kathy D. Everleth

Copy Editor: Kathryn A. Cressman

Art Director: Darlene Schneck

Cover Designer: Kristen Morgan Downey

Interior and Layout Designer: Faith Hague

Interior Illustrator: Narda Lebo

Manufacturing Coordinators: Brenda Miller, Jodi Schaffer, Patrick T. Smith

Office Manager: Roberta Mulliner

Office Staff: Julie Kehs, Suzanne Lynch

Rodale Health and Fitness Books

Vice President and Editorial Director: Debora T. Yost

Executive Editor: Neil Wertheimer

Design and Production Director: Michael Ward

Director of Product Marketing–Membership Programs: Robert Keppel

Research Manager: Ann Gossy Yermish

Copy Manager: Lisa D. Andruscavage

Production Manager: Robert V. Anderson Jr.

Associate Studio Manager: Thomas P. Aczel

Manufacturing Managers: Eileen F. Bauder, Mark Krahforst

Contents

Part 2
Boost Your Immune Power

Part 3
The Rewards of Simple Living

Part 4

Natural Weight Control

Part 5

Feel Your Mental Best

Part 6

Break Free from Pain

Part 7

Achieving Optimum Health: A Woman's Guide

Home Remedies

Part 8
Achieving Optimum Health: A Man's Guide

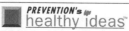

PREVENTION's *by*
healthy ideas™

For the best interactive guide to healthy active living,
visit our Web site at **www.healthyideas.com**

Introduction

If you have a look at the table of contents in this book—as you probably have by now—you'll notice that all eight parts begin with a short introduction called "Making Sense of It All."

How *do* we make sense of all the fresh news on health? How can we keep up with all the information on weight loss and nutrition—the controversy over high-protein diets, the "super staples" that belong in every kitchen, the news that an overload of iron could be making you tired? How do we make sense of all the information about women's health? What's the "designer estrogen" that can reduce the rate of osteoporosis? Should women be eating certain foods if they're on the Pill? And what about the issues that make men think twice about their health—not just impotence but also thrombosis, diverticulitis, knee pain, neck pain, and colon cancer?

We're all aware of the surge of interest in alternative medicine, but how do we make sense of the new "herbal elixirs" that are on the market—St.-John's-wort, ginkgo, valerian, feverfew? Can they really help relieve pain, boost energy, or fight depression?

Or the new initiative to simplify our lives—does it really make sense? Is "simplifying" the most logical avenue to relieving stress, improving relationships, and creating the kind of balance that allows us to enjoy and enhance a healthy lifestyle?

No doubt, you know something about these developments, but what you've heard to date may be more confusing than enlightening. We'd all like to have a personal health guidance counselor who could tell us exactly what health news is reliable, important, and relevant to our lives and our health.

As much as any book can be, that's what the 1999 edition of *Natural Healing Remedies* is to you—a personal health guidance counselor. At *Prevention* magazine and *Prevention* Health Books, we keep very careful track of every discovery and development on the health front. And our health-information tracking system is literally turned on 24 hours a day. What you find in this book is the direct result of a full year of that tracking system working full steam ahead.

To be good health guidance counselors, the editors of *Prevention* realize that we have to do far more than gather journal articles or analyze research reports. We try to get to the bottom of things. We turn to top experts in health and ask them to tell us exactly how these new findings and new developments apply to ordinary people like us.

While we're investigating, we also cast a very wide net. We know the power of nutrition as a way to prevent disease and improve health, so we keep track of every development on the nutrition front. We realize that groundbreaking research into the territory of mind-body healing is being done, so we're constantly asking researchers how people can make stress relief, meditation, and spirituality a bigger part of their lives. We see extraordinary new gains being made in women's health care, so we're constantly asking how these findings can be applied immediately to help women avoid breast cancer, prevent bone loss, ease their way through menopause, and dodge the risk of heart attack. We hear that there's a special compound found in tomatoes that can reduce the risk of prostate cancer, and on behalf of all men, we ask the researchers to tell us more. We hear about conventional and alternative techniques to fight pain.

All this inquiry and digging goes on week after week, month after month, and all with a single purpose: to deliver clear, practical, usable information into the hands of our readers.

In fact, you're the very reader we've had in mind all along. Of course, you have your own personal current health concerns—and, no doubt, you're also concerned about the health of your spouse, your family, or your friends. Perhaps there are particular concerns that are nagging you now or possible health problems that you can see on the horizon. While we can't guess exactly what those are, we do know that there's a great deal of information in this book that can help you.

The information that you find here is up-to-date, practical, easy to locate, and authoritative. You'll find many points of view—from medical doctors and alternative practitioners, proponents of diets and advocates of weight loss, leading scientific researchers and people who put research into practice. But diversity doesn't mean confusion. Turn anywhere in this book, and you'll surely find what you need to make sense of it all—the means and methods that you can adopt today to promise yourself a happier, healthier, longer life.

Edward Claflin
Senior Managing Editor
Prevention Health Books

part 1

Mother Nature's Medicine Chest

Making Sense of It All

I n this age of accelerated discovery, medical research is hitting a mother lode. Designer estrogens. Radical new cancer treatments. Viagra. Fortunately, the field of natural healing is having a heyday too. Prompted by consumer demand, more and more researchers are searching for cures in nature—and making unprecedented discoveries about the healing power of foods, supplements, herbs, exercise, and other lifestyle factors.

Vitamin E leads the list of natural remedies. Published studies suggest that this vitamin can help people with diabetes, improve immunity in older folks, prevent colon cancer, and protect against Alzheimer's disease and Parkinson's disease. All this, on top of its role as an antioxidant that fights specific cancers and heart disease. Pretty amazing stuff.

"Eat to live" is another message that's coming out loud and clear. Researchers report that a healthy, low-fat diet can dramatically reduce blood pressure–related heart attacks and strokes. In fact, the results are as good as those that you get with prescription drugs and don't require cutting salt intake or eliminating alcohol. And, say the researchers, you can begin to see blood pressure coming down within just two weeks. That's astounding.

Even more studies on specific healing foods are cropping up in medical journals these days. From green tea to grape seed and from tomatoes to tofu, the research is ripe with promise.

Herbs, too, are finally getting the scientific respect they deserve. *Prevention* advisors and top herb experts report on natural products to keep on hand to soothe everyday health problems. Have a nagging cough or upset stomach? Battling a bout with the blues? There's a home remedy for you. And don't miss the experts' list of the top 10 herbs worth buying, which begins on page 41, plus essential info on how to be an informed herb consumer.

Read on to learn about all this and more of today's leading news in natural healing.

Positive Action Plans

Breakthroughs in Natural Healing: Use Them to Change Your Life for the Better

In this fast-paced age, one year can yield a remarkable crop of major medical advances. We went to the country's top doctors—*Prevention* magazine's advisory board—to help us pick the breakthroughs that are most likely to change your life. Each works in a different way, but all may improve your health and well-being. Here's the lowdown on the high-lights—and how to use them wisely.

The Miracle Supplement

Vitamin E is the big story in nutrition. "We've gleaned more and more information on the benefits of E as an antioxidant that fights specific cancers, cardiovascular disease, and even Alzheimer's disease," says Bernadine Healy, M.D., dean of the College of Medicine at Ohio State University in Columbus, former head of the National Institutes of Health, and a *Prevention* advisor on women and heart disease.

There are studies suggesting that E can help people with the following conditions.

Diabetes. Two big findings: A small study of 36 people found that blood sugar levels fell significantly for those who were taking 800 international units (IU) of the supplement. Another study of 88 men at Tulane University in New Orleans linked low levels of vitamin E with the impotence that afflicts more than 50 percent of men with diabetes, which suggests that raising levels could help resolve that problem.

Colon cancer. A study of the diets of 645 hospital patients found that men with the highest intakes of vitamin E had about a 75 percent lower risk of adenomas (a precursor of colon cancer) than men with the lowest intakes.

Parkinson's disease. In the Netherlands, investigators studied the relationship between the antioxidant E and Parkinson's disease. They were intrigued by the idea that cell damage caused by free radicals (end products of various oxidation processes in the body) plays a large part in Parkinson's disease. High levels of E were linked to a low incidence of Parkinson's in the 5,300-plus group of people, leading researchers to conclude that the vitamin could have a protective effect.

Alzheimer's disease. Working on the same theory—that free radicals damage nerve cells—scientists at Columbia University in New York City and other centers gave high doses (2,000 IU) of E to 341 people with midstage Alzheimer's. The vitamin seemed to slow deterioration by 25 percent, mainly in the ability to do everyday tasks like dress, cook, and eat. And it delayed entrance to nursing homes by an average of seven months. Memory and comprehension didn't improve, but the evidence of benefit was strong enough to compel the American Psychiatric Association to include a recommendation for vitamin E use in its latest Alzheimer's guidelines.

Age-related impaired immune systems. Pneumonia and the flu are prime killers of the elderly. So researchers at Tufts University in Medford, Massachusetts and at Harvard and Boston Universities supplemented the diets of 88 people over the age of 65 with vitamin E to see if it improved immunity. Judging from the skin sensitivity that indicates immune response, they found that immunity improved by 65 percent when this group got optimal doses of vitamin E. Researchers also observed a sixfold increase in antibodies against one infectious disease they tested for, hepatitis B.

The Diet That Disarms High Blood Pressure

Researchers at some of the nation's most prominent medical schools, including Harvard Medical School, Johns Hopkins University School of Medicine in Baltimore, and Duke University School of Medicine in Durham, North Carolina, developed and tested a diet that they say could quickly reduce blood pressure–related heart disease in the United States by about 15 percent and spare one-fourth of the people who have strokes from getting them—if everyone adopted it.

The diet is pretty basic: low-fat foods (about 27 percent fat) that include 8 to 10 servings a day of fruits and vegetables. (One serving is one medium apple, ½ cup of cut-up fruit, 1 cup of leafy greens, or ½ cup of other vegetables, cooked or raw.) It also includes almost three servings of low-fat dairy foods. (One dairy serving is a 1-cup size.) The diet itself may not be so remarkable, but the results are as good as those achieved with drugs. People with normal blood pressure who followed it (almost 500 men) lowered blood pressure by a healthy average of 8½ points. That shaves an average 5½ points off the top (systolic) number and 3 points off the bottom (diastolic) number. People with hypertension (high blood pressure) lowered their systolic number by 11 points and their diastolic by 5½ points—all without following the standard prescriptions of cutting salt intake and eliminating alcohol. Even more astounding, the diet began lowering blood pressure within two weeks. Even the researchers themselves were surprised, says Dr. Healy.

How does the diet work? Scientists speculate that the much-larger-than-normal dose of nutrients—antioxidants, vitamins, minerals, and so on—coming from the high amounts of produce and low-fat dairy products helps keep blood pressure down. But don't expect supplements to substitute for a change in your eating habits. A single nutrient by itself won't lower your blood pressure, especially when it's combined with an unhealthy, high-fat diet. Whole, nutritious foods are what count.

The New Diabetes Rules

Sixteen million of us have diabetes, but half of us don't know it. By the time it's diagnosed, our hearts, blood vessels, and kidneys may have paid a price. Recently, the American Diabetes Association (ADA) issued three lifesaving proclamations: The organization revised the definition of the disease to help detect it earlier; it identified a way to spot diabetes while you may still be able to stifle it; and it told us when and how often to screen for the disease's mute beginnings.

Let's back up. The key to diabetes is the hormone insulin, which clears the bloodstream of glucose and enables body cells to take in this blood sugar as nourishment. People with Type I diabetes, who are usually diagnosed when they're children, lack the ability to produce insulin, and they must deal with the disease by getting daily injections of the hormone. With Type II diabetes, which is more likely to be undiagnosed and usually strikes middle-aged people (hence its other name, adult-onset diabetes), either your body doesn't make enough insulin to service your cells, or it uses the insulin that you do make inefficiently, or both. In either kind of diabetes, without sufficient insulin, blood sugar piles up in blood vessels all over your body and ruins them. Consequently, diabetes is a major cause of heart disease, stroke, blindness, and kidney failure.

Type II diabetes may creep up slowly and is considered more preventable than Type I. Most of Type II diabetes comes from putting on weight around the middle. Fortunately, the ADA's new threshold numbers will help you take preventive action more quickly. The new glucose figure that defines diabetes is 126 milligrams per deciliter (mg/dl) of blood (down from 140). Blood sugar levels from 110 to 125 mg/dl are now flagged as a condition called impaired fasting glucose. Sticking to a sensible, low-fat diet and exercising regularly may help prevent the monster from even showing its face and may keep you healthier longer. "Lowering blood sugar lowers bad blood fats and the heart attack rate," says *Prevention* heart disease advisor William Castelli, M.D., medical director of the Framingham, Massachusetts, Cardiovascular Institute and former director of the Framingham Heart Study.

How often to test? The ADA says every three years after the age of 45. The test is cheap and simple—a fasting plasma glucose (FPG) test. People with risk factors for the disease (the big ones: family history of the disease, high blood pressure, lack of exercise, being overweight) need to start screening even earlier. As it is now, doctors don't diagnose diabetes in many people until they have had it for seven or more years, and that's too much time for the disease to attack blood vessels and organs.

Dental Floss Could Save Your Life

The past year uncovered one of the most unlikely ways to prevent heart disease: Keep your gums healthy. A large study at the University of North Carolina in Chapel Hill further validated what much other research had already hinted at: Periodontal disease is a risk factor for heart disease.

So what's the connection between your heart and your mouth? The pockets formed when sick gums pull away from teeth "have one of the highest concentrations of bacteria in the body," answers *Prevention* dental advisor Dominick DePaola, D.D.S., Ph.D., president of Baylor College of Dentistry in Dallas. Gum disease is an infectious disease, and the infection can result in bacteria being pumped into the bloodstream, which may damage the heart walls or valves. The bacteria may also cause the release of those cruel clotting factors that can spur heart attacks and strokes. What you can do is keep up your flossing, which helps stop gum disease. "The head is connected to the rest of the body. So when you prevent disease in one place, like the mouth, it has all kinds of important consequences on overall health and well-being," says Dr. DePaola. Sometimes life really is simple.

Estrogen without the Worry

Finally, there's a new set of estrogens that beef up your bones and help your heart but don't increase your risk of breast or uterine cancer. The first one—raloxifene—hit the market in 1998.

"Designer" estrogens should clear up a lot of the hormonal murk that women wade through at menopause and afterward. Many women can't or won't take hormone replacement therapy (HRT) because of its side effects (mainly, bleeding) or because they are concerned about breast cancer. The women who do take HRT do so to relieve menopausal symptoms and to protect themselves from heart disease and bone-thinning osteoporosis. Raloxifene, like regular estrogen, may actually build bone (not just keep it stable). In fact, during the final Phase III clinical trial of the drug, which involved 12,000 women, the hormone increased bone mass by 2 to 3 percent in the hip and spine sites of severe fractures in older women with thinned bones. That ability to fight osteoporosis spurred the Food and Drug Administration (FDA) to fast-track the drug for approval.

The proper name for designer estrogens is "selective estrogen receptor modulators," or SERMs. They work by attaching to estrogen receptors in the cells. The marriage unlocks the cell's DNA so it can activate genes that do things including lay down bone cells. But because their shape is a little different from that of natural estrogens, SERMs don't turn on the cells that build breast or uterine tissue. In fact, raloxifene was first developed to treat breast cancer, so experts think that it may even have a preventive effect on the disease. Raloxifene won't make other forms of HRT obsolete. It doesn't reduce—and may increase—heavy-duty hot flashes. "So for women right in the midst of menopause who have lots of symptoms, this is probably not the right drug. I think what will happen as women pass through menopause is that they'll start on HRT if they're symptomatic and then make the transition to raloxifene," says Brian Walsh, M.D., director of the menopause clinic at Brigham and Women's Hospital in Boston. But women who don't like the bleeding that can come with HRT and don't have hot flashes, but who want to safeguard their heart and bones, can skip estrogen and progestin and proceed straight to raloxifene.

The Shortcut to Fitness

The mandate that our bodies give us to either work out or fall apart has gotten a lot easier to obey.

Several studies found that we only need to strength train (lift weights or use bands or machines) twice a week, not three times. They also showed that one set of exercises—say, 10 to 12 biceps curls—is as beneficial as three sets of 10 to 12 repetitions. That pared-down minimum won't turn us into Arnolds or Chers, but it will develop muscles, reduce fat, and build stronger bones.

Prevention's strength-training advisor, Wayne Westcott, Ph.D., who is strength consultant to the YMCA of the USA and author of *Strength Training Past 50*, has been studying how to squeeze strength training into people's lives. One of his investigations involved 1,132 people and was the largest of its kind so far.

The study focused on body composition. "That's what most of the middle-aged and senior adults we train are interested in," says Dr. Westcott. "You know, how do I look? What's my muscle gain and fat loss?"

Dr. Westcott and his colleagues found that "across the board, in percentage of body fat, muscle gain, and weight loss, twice-a-week training produced 90 percent as much benefit in terms of fat loss and muscle gain as three-times-a-week training. It wasn't exactly 100 percent, but it was very high."

The Center for Exercise Science at the University of Florida, Gainesville, also studied the question of training sets. They found that one set "produced exactly the same benefits in 14 weeks as three sets in people who were beginners at weight training," says Dr. Westcott.

"So this is the way to go if you're just starting out or if you're limited on time," he says. Here's some extra motivation: When Dr. Westcott did a study similar to the University of Florida's study on the number of training sets necessary for fitness, he discovered that the people who were doing only one set of 10 repetitions in their exercise programs gained an average 2½ pounds of muscle and lost 4½ pounds of fat in two months.

Stock Your Fridge with Nature's Best Medicines

Laboratory scientists constantly grab headlines for cooking up new miraculous medicines. We, too, cook up miracle medicines—daily, in our kitchens, and to much less fanfare. We work with nature's most powerful healing and health-promoting potions.

These are medicines that for the most part are found in supermarkets and are never tough to swallow. It's easy to forget these champs when they become background noise in the supermarket hype of "new" and "lite." Don't let them get eclipsed. Beneath their everyday exterior, these foods are health-giving powerhouses. Each made it onto our list because it has the double-dip advantage of being tasty as well as able to prevent more than one health problem. Put all of these foods in your grocery basket every week, and you'll get compliments on dinner. And you'll be around to get those compliments for a long, long time.

The Champion Crucifer

Broccoli speaks many languages and is a welcome item in cuisines throughout the world—steamed, stir-fried, blanched, baked, or raw. But it's not always the most wanted veggie in the West, and that's unfortunate.

True, broccoli may not have won any presidential medals, but it has heroic potential to fight today's major diseases.

- It's stuffed with compounds that may block cancer. One of these steps up the body's production of a weak estrogen. This weak version seems to replace the "real" estrogen that's implicated in breast cancer.
- It offers heart protection through vitamin C. This antioxidant vitamin helps keep arteries elastic and helps prevent blood from getting sludgy. A single serving of broccoli gives us 97 percent of our Daily Value (DV) of vitamin C.
- It contains glutathione, which may reduce the risks of arthritis, diabetes, and heart disease as well as bolster the immune system, lower cholesterol, lower blood pressure, and keep people at a healthy weight, according to a small study.

- It helps guard against cataracts and the leading cause of blindness over age 65—macular degeneration—because it's rich in beta-carotene and its cousin, lutein.

How much do I need? The amount of broccoli that you need to prevent disease hasn't been quantified. But Walter C. Willett, M.D., Dr.P.H., chairman of the department of nutrition at Harvard School of Public Health, advises you to put it on your grocery list now—in any quantity. Broccoli can definitely be a contributor to your total score of five fruits and vegetables. Just ½ cup is considered a serving and delivers an impressive 2 grams of fiber.

The Potent, Redolent Clove

Garlic wards off many a bad guy, and you needn't wear it around your neck. Eat it. Any way you can. There may be foods more medicinally potent than garlic, but few are as loved as this.

One of garlic's most proven benefits is its ability to cut cholesterol, says *Prevention* advisor and America's foremost expert on herbs and plant-derived medicine Varro E. Tyler, Ph.D. Sc.D., dean emeritus of the Purdue University School of Pharmacy and Pharmacal Sciences, distinguished professor emeritus of pharmacognosy, and author of more than 270 scientific articles and 18 books, including *The Honest Herbal*. It also acts like aspirin, keeping blood from clumping and sticking to artery walls.

Garlic has an antibacterial effect similar to penicillin. In fact, one source suggests that garlic was the antibacterial drug of choice until penicillin was discovered in 1928. Eating this pungent herb may help you fight a strep throat—as long as you don't use it instead of antibiotics for serious infections. Garlic is an antioxidant and, in test-tube and animal studies, shows promise in preventing colon and breast cancers.

Allicin, which is quickly broken down into various active compounds, seems to be the main medicine at work here, says Dr. Tyler.

How much do I need? For heart-protective effects, eat one clove daily. Aged, cooked, raw, or powdered? Overall, studies seem to indicate that any and all garlic intake is probably good for us in some way.

The Queen of Beans

Kidney beans, those staples of hearty winter chili, boast the highest, healthiest fiber mix of any member of the legume family—and are especially high in heart-protecting folate, too.

Counting Beans

Kidney beans are tops for soluble fiber and tie with lima beans for total fiber. Other beans supply healthy amounts as well. Here are the measures of soluble fiber and total fiber per half-cup servings of cooked beans.

	Soluble Fiber (g.)	Total Fiber (g.)
Kidney beans	2.8	6.9
Lima beans	2.7	6.9
Cranberry beans	2.7	5.4
Black beans	2.4	6.1
Navy beans	2.2	6.5
Pinto beans	1.9	5.9
Great Northern beans	1.4	5.0
Chickpeas	1.3	4.3

Part of their healing power comes from their 7 grams of filling fiber per half-cup serving. Of that, 2.8 grams is cholesterol-lowering soluble fiber. That adds up to dips in the risks of heart disease, stroke, and colon cancer.

If that's not enough, beans—kidney and otherwise—are such good medicine that doctors prescribe them to people who have diabetes (along with other high-fiber, complex carbohydrates) because they're digested slowly, helping maintain low blood sugar and normalizing troublesome insulin levels, says *Prevention* advisor James W. Anderson, M.D., professor of medicine and clinical nutrition at the University of Kentucky College of Medicine in Lexington.

Kidney beans are high in folate, the new superstar nutrient that may help keep blood levels of homocysteine low. (High levels are now considered a risk factor for heart disease.) Folate is also important in preventing birth defects. A half-cup serving provides 114 micrograms of folate, more than a quarter of our required DV.

Beans are heart-protective in one more way: They contain potent antioxidants known as polyphenolics. In test-tube studies, polyphenolics worked better than vitamin C in keeping fat in the blood from oxidizing and initiating the formation of artery-clogging sludge. Human research is now under way, reports Dr. Anderson.

How much do I need? Aim for 1½ cups of cooked beans daily. That's enough to lower cholesterol and provide the other health benefits, says Dr. Anderson.

Dairy Dearest

Leave the mustache on your lip, refill your glass, and join us in a toast. Milk—the fat-free variety—is just about the best food source of calcium around.

Milk helps prevent osteoporosis (brittle bones), which affects at least half of all American women over age 50. Calcium is the bone builder in milk, and the vitamin D in milk helps us absorb the calcium.

In addition, fat-free milk, combined with a low-fat diet rich in fruits and vegetables, has been shown to lower blood pressure as well as any single prescription drug does, says *Prevention* advisor Judith Stern, R.D., Sc.D., professor of nutrition and internal medicine at the University of California, Davis. The calcium, potassium, and magnesium in milk help with that.

Milk consumption also has been associated with a lower risk of kidney stones. That's because calcium binds oxalate in the large bowel so that less is absorbed. Oxalate is what causes most kidney stones, says Dr. Willett, whose Harvard group has published two papers on this topic.

How much do I need? Each eight-ounce glass of fat-free milk contains 300 milligrams of calcium. Women under 50 and men under 65 need 1,000 milligrams of calcium per day. If you're older, up that to 1,500 milligrams. It can be difficult to meet all of your calcium needs with milk, but it's a smart way to get at least halfway to your daily requirement.

The Sunny Side of Citrus

There's no better way to find concentrated sunshine in the dark, short days of winter. Peel and bite into an orange. This is the sweetest medicine around.

"Oranges are probably one of the best creations of the universe," says James Cerda, M.D., director of the nutrition research laboratory at the University of Florida College of Medicine in Gainesville.

This juicy fruit is chock-full of vitamins, nutrients, and soluble fibers that may ward off colds, lower cholesterol, build bones, prevent kidney stones, lessen risk of colon cancer, and speed recovery from heart attack. The phytochemicals that it contains may even be able to help fight breast cancer.

Vitamin C is a major player in the benefits that oranges give you, and they are robust with this nutrient. Each average orange packs 70 milligrams of C, almost 110 percent of our DV. In addition, oranges are ripe with folate, glutathione, and potassium citrate, which has been shown to help dissolve kidney stones and is an important ingredient in sports drinks. (It keeps electrolytes in balance when you're sweating a lot.)

How much do I need? Get at least an orange a day. Two would be better, says Dr. Cerda. Eat the whole orange (sans peel) to get the pulp and fiber. Don't skip the albedo—the mild-tasting white material just under the peel and comprising the cord at the center of the orange—it's full of clot-fighting substances called flavonoids. Juice conveys fewer benefits but is especially good when you're working out or sweating a lot in heat and humidity.

To pick the best, look for firm, heavy oranges with bright skin. Avoid lightweight oranges (which are probably light on juice) and those with dull, dry skin or a spongy texture—indicators of aging.

King Fish

Salmon is king when it comes to netting the myriad benefits of fish oil. The fish story is this: All fish have fats called omega-3 fatty acids, but salmon is one of the richest sources. And omega-3's are turning out to be major players in the prevention of heart problems and maybe in controlling inflammatory problems like arthritis.

Omega-3's may guard against heart attacks. One study of 44,895 men found that guys who favored food with fins had a 26 percent lower risk of death from coronary disease than those who chose to forgo fish. In another study, people who ate the equivalent of just one serving of salmon weekly had half the risk of cardiac arrest as those who ate none.

It appears that these "good" fats work by assuring the orderly inflow of calcium, sodium, and other charged particles into each heart cell, which helps ensure a steady, strong beat.

Salmon also reels in one of the shadiest characters implicated in rheumatoid arthritis inflammation, leukotriene B_4. Scientists can measure a significant drop when fish oil is added to the diet.

Fish oil may also lessen severe menstrual cramping and other menstrual symptoms (though only one study so far shows convincing relief), and may even stave off depression.

How much do I need? A single three-ounce serving of baked salmon provides 10 times the amount of omega-3's that the typical American gets in a week. Eat at least one serving weekly. For menstrual cramp relief, you need to eat even more—four to six ounces daily. To relieve rheumatoid arthritis symptoms, step up intake to at least one serving daily, or ask your doctor about supplementing with fish oil capsules. One tip: All species of salmon contain fish oil, although smoked salmon does not. (During smoking, much of the fat drips out.)

Soy Rewards

Tofu. It almost sounds like an insult, and too many of us have shunned it as though it were. But this simple, palatable, easy-to-use, and oh-so-versatile soybean derivative is nothing short of a superfood when it comes to our health.

Tofu is mild and light-bodied and represents "one of our very best food choices," says Dr. Anderson. Soy's potential health benefits are sweeping, he adds. Topping the list is major heart protection. Its choles-terol-lowering effect has been shown in 37 studies.

Smart Ways to Slip Tofu into Your Diet

A daily serving of tofu may sound like a lot. It's not. Really. Here are some ways to slip it into your diet.

- Blend it in a shake or smoothie.
- Crumble it on a salad.
- Chuck chunks into soups, stews, chili, and marinara sauce.
- Slice it like cheese for a sandwich.
- Blend it into dips, dressings, custards, and puddings.
- Drink calcium-fortified, low-fat soy milk—with about 20 milligrams of isoflavones and only 2.5 grams of fat per one-cup serving. For a treat, wash down some White Wave Chocolate Silk—a smooth chocolate soy milk.

Tofu is soybean curd, and soybeans are the richest source by far of isoflavones, a plant version of estrogen. This may be important in some of the other protective roles that tofu is believed to play a part in, such as soothing menopause symptoms, preventing osteoporosis, and reducing breast cancer risk. Isoflavones are also known kidney protectors. And there's evidence that soy may help reduce the risk of prostate cancer and possibly colon cancer, as well.

How much do I need? For now, most soy researchers recommend 30 to 50 milligrams of isoflavones per day. That's about what the average daily intake is in Asia, where tofu is thought of as comfort food. (A half-cup serving of tofu has 35 milligrams of isoflavones.) Cultivating a taste for tofu is easy; it can be added to almost anything.

Good Health, Italian-Style

Tomato sauce beats ripe tomatoes to a pulp when it comes to being a nutritional strongman. Here's where cooking really counts and makes nature's best even better.

Tomato sauce, especially when cooked in even the tiniest bit of olive oil, seems to be a good guard against prostate cancer. Some evidence suggests that it may protect against colon, esophageal, and stomach cancers, as well. Plus, tomato sauce may even contribute to agility as we age (though the connection comes only from a small study).

The hot nutrient here is lycopene, an antioxidant that's found in ap-

Put the Squeeze on Your Tomatoes

To squeeze the full dose of usable lycopene from a tomato, you need to cook the tomato in oil. (By the way, lycopene is what makes tomatoes red; green tomatoes have less of it.) A tiny bit of oil will do, says Edward Giovannucci, M.D., Sc.D., of Harvard Medical School, and heart-healthy olive oil is just fine.

The lycopene is absorbed into the oil as the heat of cooking breaks down the tomato's cell walls. How big of a boost can this cook up? In experiments, people eating tomato sauce cooked with oil got roughly 10 times more lycopene into their systems as did people drinking processed tomato juice containing the same amount of lycopene.

preciable amounts in few other fruits and vegetables. Lycopene may prevent cancer from developing. Molecules called free radicals are thought to beat up innocent cells and force them to become cancerous, but lycopene may mop up these radicals before they do harm. The nutrient may even be twice as potent a free radical fighter as strongman beta-carotene, says Edward Giovannucci, M.D., Sc.D., of Harvard Medical School.

How much do I need? A few servings each week, but don't eat a lot of fattening cheese-and-pepperoni pizza to get your quota. Salsas and spaghetti sauce count.

The Clear Choice

We bathe in it, relax in it, exercise in it—and should be guzzling it. Our bodies are mostly made of it. And it's a wonder medicine. H_2O.

One thing water won't do is set you back a pretty penny, unless you buy it in designer-shaped bottles. "It's the original no-calorie beverage," says Dr. Stern.

Water is the elixir required by every cell for optimum health. Getting enough water helps stave off the fatigue and muscle cramping that result from even minor dehydration, maintains body temperature, helps prevent kidney stone formation, and keeps the skin looking healthy. And, in a surprise finding of a large study, drinking more than five glasses of water a day seemed to slice women's colon cancer risks in half compared with those who drank fewer than two glasses a day.

Our bodies need water. Without it, we droop like thirsty houseplants. Each cell's chemical, mineral, nutrient, and vitamin balance depends upon just the right balance of fluid.

How much do I need? Your total fluid intake should be 48 to 64 ounces (that's six to eight glasses) a day—more if you're very active.

Can a Handful of Grapes a Day Keep the Doctor Away?

Herb expert and Prevention *advisor Varro E. Tyler, Ph.D., Sc.D., shares his scientific perspective on a popular folk cure passed along "the grapevine."*

Another Grape Product

Resveratrol is not the only component of grapes that is believed to have disease-fighting capabilities. Grape seed extract, which contains no resveratrol at all, has been marketed in the United States for several years as an herbal supplement. It contains a mixture of complex phenolic compounds, the names of which are incomprehensible to everyone but organic chemists—and are even confusing to them.

European studies have shown a potential value of one group of grape seed compounds—procyanidins—in treating vascular disorders such as fragile capillaries and inadequate circulation in the veins. The compounds are thought to bind to the elastic fibers of the capillaries, making them less likely to break down with aging. (This has never been proved in the United States to the satisfaction of the Food and Drug Administration.)

In addition, procyanidins act as antioxidants, or scavengers of free radicals, and thus are believed to help prevent some types of cancer and atherosclerosis that tend to occur with aging. But this preventive activity alone was not enough to account for the purported anti-cancer activity of grapes as touted in such folkloric treatments as the grape cure (see below). The cancer-fighting chore is where resveratrol appears to play a significant role.

The recent discovery that a compound present in the skin of grapes may help prevent cancer just proves the old adage "What goes around, comes around." Way back in 1927, a South African naturopath named Johanna Brandt came to the United States to promote her so-called grape cure for cancer. Details of her regimen were first published in 1928 in a 220-page paperback entitled *The Grape Cure*.

In my numerous visits to secondhand bookstores over the years, I had often seen dusty copies of this volume on the shelves in the folk-medicine sections. But I must admit that I had never purchased one, because the subject just seemed too far out. However, the recent publicity on the anti-cancer properties of grapes finally prompted me to invest $2.00 in a copy.

The Grape Diet

Basically, the treatment involved initial fasting for two or three days, followed by an exclusive diet of grapes eaten every two hours beginning at 8:00 A.M. and ending at 8:00 P.M. Any variety of grapes could be used—purple, green, white, or blue—and somewhere between one and four pounds were to be consumed each day. The whole grapes, including both skin and seeds, were to be chewed thoroughly prior to swallowing. One can't help wondering just how many people actually followed this drastic regimen. Not many, I hope. No scientific studies have ever proved that a diet of grapes can cure cancer. And if you followed such a restricted diet for more than a few days, you'd be on the road to malnutrition. After about a month or so, Dr. Brandt allowed other raw foods, but grapes—and later grape juice—remained an integral part of the six-month cure.

Without any scientific evidence, Dr. Brandt simply believed that "elements in the grape break down malignant growths." But we had to wait 50 years for research to reveal a compound that supports her hunch.

Preventing Heart Attacks and More

The anti-cancer element appears to be resveratrol, a simple compound found in grapes that was initially touted for a role in preventing heart disease. Animal studies have shown that resveratrol lowers cholesterol, inhibits platelet aggregation (thereby making blood more slippery), and prevents blood clots.

Resveratrol has been detected in 72 different plant species, including mulberries and peanuts, as well as in grape juice and red wine. The relatively high quantities in the grape skins are thought to help the plant resist fungal infections.

Recently, a group of scientists at the University of Illinois at Chicago, led by John M. Pezzuto, Ph.D., described test-tube and animal studies that showed resveratrol prevents cancer. Their preliminary tests showed that resveratrol may interfere with the development of cancer in three different ways: by blocking the action of cancer-causing agents, by inhibiting the development and growth of tumors, and by causing precancerous cells to revert to normal.

Before hailing grapes as the miracle food/drug of this century, more studies are needed. At the moment, it's not known if results will be similar in humans or how much resveratrol is needed to produce beneficial effects.

My best advice at this point, if you want to take advantage of the potential benefits, would be to add a glass of grape juice or some grapes to your diet. Grape jams, purees, and raisins may also provide small amounts of this potential anti-cancer compound. Although resveratrol occurs in red wine, and with lesser amounts in white and rose wines as well, the long-term consumption of large amounts of alcohol may produce adverse health effects.

In view of the aggressive nature of the American dietary supplement industry, I suspect that in a relatively short time, products containing specific amounts of resveratrol will be appearing in stores (with the resveratrol either obtained from grape skins or produced synthetically). It may even be combined with other suspected disease-preventing compounds in grapes. When that occurs, remember that the studies are still preliminary.

The whole 1927 grape cure/1997 resveratrol scenario causes me to wonder how many other examples of folk medicine are out there waiting to be validated—or possibly, invalidated—by modern scientific and clinical methodologies.

Your New Guide to Supplements

They line the shelves in health food stores like little soldiers. Small brown bottles. Lab-coat white jars. Some you recognize, like calcium, vitamin E, and beta-carotene. But what about that other stuff, like CoQ_{10}, alpha-lipoic acid, blue-green algae, and colloidal minerals. What are they for?

As you push your cart through this paradise of promised health, you have to wonder: What do I really need for a fit, long life? Nearly every day, you read a news story touting the benefits of one supplement or another. And nearly every day, it seems, a new name appears on the "hot" list. Health food stores offer a staggering bounty of possibilities. No wonder you're confused.

Well, to help clear up some of that confusion, the editors of *Preven-*

Prevention–NBC Today
Pulse of America Survey

Do you take a multivitamin each morning? If not, maybe you should. If you already do, you're in good company. Nearly two-thirds of Americans supplement their diets with vitamins, minerals, or other products, according to a *Prevention–NBC Today Weekend Edition* survey.*

44% of American adults take multis.

38% take individual vitamins such as E or C.

22% take individual minerals such as calcium or magnesium.

Fewer than **4%** of the nation's adults take nonnutrient supplements such as shark cartilage, melatonin, DHEA, or alpha-lipoic acid.

And, folks aren't waiting until they're sick or stressed to supplement—smart move!

79% of users take supplements daily to ensure good health.

53% of users say that vitamins and minerals can help prevent common illnesses, but supplements are greatly underestimated in their disease-preventing abilities. Only **28%** of users expect to ward off serious diseases such as heart disease.

Still, many people are missing out on the benefits.

38% of Americans don't take any supplements.

Why not?

78% say they get what they need from food. (The truth: it's difficult to get optimum levels of many vital nutrients from food alone without eating too many calories.)

24% say they don't know what to take.

22% say they cost too much.

20% say their doctors don't recommend it.

18% think they're unsafe.

Results are based on telephone interviews with a nationally representative sample of 797 adults age 18 or older, conducted from January 9 to 12, 1998. Margin of error: +/- 4.0 percentage points.

tion hunted down experts, reviewed studies, and got the goods on many of the nutrients and other nonherbal supplements—which range from sex hormones to dressed-up pond scum—that you may have heard about. Here are a few that you may want to toss in your shopping cart as well as a few to steer clear of.

Put These in Your Basket

You exercise. You eat well. But you just want a little extra insurance to help keep disease at bay. Since you're unlikely to get optimum levels of all the essential nutrients from food alone—you'd have to eat too many calories—you're wise to think about supplementing. First, experts recommend picking up a good multivitamin/mineral supplement, plus separate supplements of calcium and vitamins C and E.

But new research is emphasizing the health benefits of three more nutrients that are often in short supply in your diet and in good multivitamins. Consider taking the following minerals as separate supplements. *Caution:* People with abnormal kidney function should check with their doctors before supplementing with minerals.

Magnesium. Single-dose multis don't go above 100 milligrams of this mineral. And the foods in which this is most abundant—whole grains, soybeans, and nuts, for example—aren't usually eaten with the regularity that would ensure adequate intake. But magnesium is important. The diseases that it could protect you from are all killers: diabetes, heart disease, high blood pressure, and osteoporosis. It may also help relieve migraines. Aim for a total of 350 milligrams from both your multi and a supplement. (More than that may cause diarrhea.)

Chromium. It's hard to get the Daily Value (DV) of 120 micrograms of chromium from food alone. Even many multis come up short. But chromium is absolutely vital in helping your body process glucose for energy. Insufficient levels of chromium may increase your risk of adult-onset diabetes, and studies suggest that 200 to 1,000 micrograms of chromium can improve your symptoms if you have the disease. But more studies on long-term supplementation still need to be done. Don't take more than 200 micrograms without checking first with your doctor.

Selenium. This antioxidant is showing great promise as a cancer fighter. One 10-year study of 1,300 people found that those who took 200-microgram supplements cut their rate of cancer overall by 39 percent and their rates of lung, prostate, and colon cancers nearly in half. Don't exceed 200 micrograms total, including the amount in your multivitamin.

Worth a Look

These nonnutrient supplements are the headline grabbers. While preliminary research looks good, they're not for everyone. Many health experts want to see more studies before recommending them.

Glucosamine and chondroitin. Your body makes these two substances to help build and protect cartilage, the shock-absorbing cushion that caps the ends of your bones. The commercial combination of the two has been touted in *The Arthritis Cure,* a best-selling book by Jason Theodosakis, M.D. Preliminary studies, mostly European, have shown that it reduces pain and slows down cartilage loss in osteoarthritis, the wear-and-tear kind of arthritis that causes aching, deteriorating joints. Alternative health practitioners and even some mainstream doctors in the United States have also reported some success with the combo.

The word *cure* is an overstatement, though. In Hendersonville, North Carolina, orthopedic surgeon Amal Das, M.D., is analyzing data from a study that he recently completed. "The combination was significantly effective for pain relief in people with mild to moderate arthritis," he says, "but not for severe arthritis."

How much: Follow label directions. You can get the two supplements either separately or as a combination. But be careful what you buy: A University of Maryland study found a few products that contained far less glucosamine or chondroitin than labels claimed. Two combination products that passed the study's quality tests were Cosamin DS and Joint Fuel. If you try them, tell your doctor. Give the supplements eight weeks to work—it often takes that long. If you don't see any improvement by then, stop using them. So far, both glucosamine and chondroitin appear safe.

Alpha-lipoic acid (ALA). A relative newcomer to the market, ALA is an antioxidant that your body normally makes on its own. It helps break down food into the energy needed by your cells. Supplementing may be helpful if you have or are at high risk for diabetes, because your energy metabolism is impaired. Preliminary studies suggest that ALA prevents the nerve damage in the lower legs that often occurs as the result of diabetes, possibly because of its protective effect on the smaller blood vessels.

Everyday Supplements

The best preventive medicine is a great diet and regular exercise. But no matter what the state of your health, it's just smart to take a multi supplement that contains 100 percent of the Daily Value (DV) for most essential vitamins and minerals. (None contains them all.) Pay particular attention to getting suggested amounts of these nutrients, which many diets shortchange, experts say.

In Your Daily Multivitamin/Mineral Supplement

Vitamin A/beta-carotene: 5,000 international units (IU)

Vitamin B_6: 2 milligrams

Vitamin D: 400 IU

Folic acid/folate: 400 micrograms

Magnesium: 100 milligrams (That's as much as you'll find in a multi; any more of this bulky mineral would turn a one-a-day supplement into a horse pill.)

Zinc: 15 milligrams

Copper: 2 milligrams

Chromium: 120 micrograms

Selenium: At least 10 micrograms (DV is 70 micrograms, but most multivitamins contain less.)

Unless you have iron-deficiency anemia, look for a multi with no iron. You probably don't need extra iron, and recent studies have linked high iron levels with increased risk of heart attack and atherosclerosis (a buildup of fatty deposits on your arteries).

Take These Every Day

You won't find the optimal dose of the following nutrients in any multi, so buy them separately.

Vitamin C: 500 milligrams a day, but you'll keep your blood better saturated if you take two 250-milligram doses spaced 12 hours apart

Vitamin E: 200 IU

Calcium: 500 to 1,000 milligrams

Guinea Pig Pills

Under the 1994 Dietary Supplement Health and Education Act, manufacturers don't have to prove that supplements work or that they're safe before selling them. The Food and Drug Administration (FDA) classifies these products as dietary supplements, not drugs. By law, drugs must meet rigorous testing standards for safety and efficacy before getting FDA approval. Yet people often use supplements as if they were drugs—to prevent or treat disease. (By the way, a supplement label that claims to prevent or treat disease is illegal.)

Don't be a guinea pig by self-prescribing the following products.

DHEA (dehydroepiandrosterone) is a weak male hormone that your body makes. Your levels drop as you grow older, so some people take the supplement to circumvent the symptoms of aging. "I've seen some noteworthy improvements in older patients' muscle mass and memory. And their depression gets better," says Alan R. Gaby, M.D., professor of nutrition at Bastyr University in Seattle. But DHEA is a steroid hormone, he warns. In theory, it could increase your risk of breast or prostate cancer. You should only use it if blood tests show that your DHEA levels are low, says Dr. Gaby. And your doctor should always monitor DHEA treatment.

Melatonin is a nonsteroidal hormone that your body makes. Your pineal gland releases it in response to darkness, so melatonin is tightly tied to your sleep/wake cycle. Normal production slows as you age. That's why supplementation can be useful for older people who have phase-shift insomnia, meaning that they fall asleep, but later than they'd like—which often leaves them exhausted the next day. Melatonin helps reset their body clocks to acceptable hours. Melatonin is also used to help ease jet lag.

Short-term use seems benign so far, although some people report odd dreams. Regular, long-term use is not recommended.

How much: The effective dosage in one recent study of people with diabetes was 800 milligrams a day for four months. No adverse effects were reported.

Coenzyme Q₁₀ (CoQ₁₀). This is another antioxidant manufactured by the body, where it goes by the name ubiquinone. This supplement claims many healing powers. Right now, however, the potential benefits

Pregnenolone is an up-and-coming supplement that you'll be seeing more of in health food stores. It's another anti-aging hormone—"a precursor to DHEA," explains Elson Haas, M.D., director of the Preventive Medical Center of Marin in San Rafael, California. Pregnenolone improved the memory of aging rodents in one study, says Dr. Gaby, but research so far is sparse and preliminary.

What is known is that both pregnenolone and DHEA increase the levels of estrogen and testosterone in your body, which means that women could grow facial hair and that men's breasts could enlarge, says Dr. Haas. "That isn't often seen with the lower amounts (5 to 10 milligrams) found in health food store products," he says. "It can happen, though."

Jerald Foote, R.D., a nutritionist in Arvada, California, recommends taking extreme caution with hormones. "Think of the care that you and your doctor take over the decision on hormone replacement therapy (HRT). Anyone taking hormone supplements is doing HRT." And due to potential risks of steroidal hormone-related cancers (of the prostate and breast), seek advice from your doctor.

Colloidal supplements sprang from the theory that minerals au naturel—combined the way that you find them in rich soil—would be the best way for your body to get them. We can't rely on fruits and vegetables for minerals, the theory goes, because bad farming practices have depleted farming soil. But this theory doesn't quite hold up to scrutiny. "Your body is used to absorbing minerals from food. (Taking colloidal supplements is) like eating soil to get your minerals," says Foote. And colloidal supplements made from so-called good earth can come with an unwanted bonus—lead, aluminum, pollutants, even arsenic. Though Foote believes that colloidal companies have started removing those things, he recommends giving colloidal supplements a wide berth.

of CoQ_{10} appear to be limited to helping you if you have or are at risk for congestive heart failure, which occurs when your heart is too weak to pump blood to your lungs and the rest of your body. It may also be good for gum disease, a leading cause of tooth loss.

How much: One study found that 150 milligrams per day protected some people with congestive heart failure (people using that amount were hospitalized 38 percent less often than people taking placebos). And 50 to 60 milligrams a day helped reverse gum disease.

Caution: While CoQ_{10} appears safe, congestive heart failure and gingivitis are not do-it-yourself diseases. They require a doctor's care.

Walk On By

Some supplements remain mysteries yet to be solved by further research. And some, based on a lack of evidence so far, don't justify the expense.

Shark cartilage. While you can't write off this tabloid supplement yet, it's too soon to start taking shark pills to ward off cancer. Promoters speculate whether shark cartilage can prevent cancer by blocking blood vessel growth in tumors, depriving them of nutrients to grow. But there are no well-controlled studies to support this. And forming new blood vessels isn't always a bad thing, points out Alan R. Gaby, M.D., professor of nutrition at Bastyr University in Seattle. It's useful when your cardio-vascular system is trying to move blood around blockages, for example, or during pregnancy or for wound healing. Dr. Gaby also doubts that popular oral supplements of shark cartilage can even make it into the bloodstream, because their active ingredient is a protein destroyed by digestion.

Blue-green algae. This supplement comes in more than 1,000 different strains that grow in lakes and oceans. The algae available as a supplement generally began life in a lake as pond scum. It does contain protein, B vitamins, and minerals, but algae leaves a lot of nutrition experts cold. You can get plenty of those same nutrients from food and a multi, notes Dr. Gaby. There have also been reports of toxicity, contamination, and illness associated with some algae.

Chromium. Theoretically, using chromium for weight loss could work, says University of Massachusetts health sciences dean and researcher Priscilla Clarkson, Ph.D. "Chromium enhances insulin action. And insulin aids fat metabolism. That means chromium could potentially burn fat. But that theory hasn't yet become fact." Studies showing that supplemental chromium takes off the pounds have been weak or inconsistent.

Chelated supplements Chelation is simply a technique for binding minerals with another substance that's supposed to enhance mineral absorption by the body. But actual studies proving better absorption are few. Specific use of the word *chelated* on a mineral supplement label is often just a marketing buzzword to make you think that it's better than the rest, says Dr. Gaby.

Sage Advice

Green Tea Extract Is Hot

Ever heard of green tea extract? It's a supplement that concentrates a cup of green tea into one capsule—and it's a product to watch. Here's why.

Green tea brims with cancer-fighters (antioxidants) that block cancer by preventing damage to cell DNA. One of these, EGCG, recently tested 100 times stronger than vitamin C and 25 times stronger than vitamin E at protecting DNA. So impressed was medicinal chemist Lester Mitscher, Ph.D., of the University of Kansas in Lawrence, an expert in changes that cause cancer, that he now takes a daily green tea extract supplement. Why not just drink tea? "As busy as I am, it's hard to set aside time to brew several cups of tea a day," Dr. Mitscher says, though he points out that we still need proof that green tea extract works.

Proof may be on the way. At the prestigious M.D. Anderson Cancer Center in Houston, they've begun testing green tea extract supplements in patients with cancer. Researchers will look for side effects (though few if any are expected) as well as possible shrinkage of tumors. Green tea inhibits many kinds of cancer in test-tube and animal studies. M.D. Anderson medical oncologist Waun Ki Hong, M.D., points out that green tea-drinkers in Japan have less cancer. And those who drink green tea and still develop cancer generally do so at an older age. Green tea is the coffee of Japan: People routinely drink two to three cups a day and often more.

Will green tea extract supplements work? Only future studies will tell. In the meantime, drink green or black tea. Though green tea has more EGCG, both have antioxidants, says Dr. Mitscher, "so drink whichever kind you like."

A New Clue to Why Fish Buoys Heart Health

There's a mysterious new risk factor for heart disease—something called Lp(a) (doctors say "ell-pee-little-a"). Especially among people under age 55, if your blood levels of Lp(a) are too high, research indicates that you're at increased risk for heart disease. "And until now, it's been frustrating to treat," says heart-health expert William Castelli, M.D., *Prevention* heart disease advisor, medical director of the Framingham, Massachusetts, Cardiovascular Institute, and former director of the Framingham Heart Study, "because nothing seems to lower it, with the possible exceptions of aspirin and red wine."

Finally, researchers looked at two groups of Bantu villagers in Tanzania. One group lives by a lake and eats mostly grains and vegetables, plus lots of fish—enough to supply three to five grams of omega-3 fatty acids per day. These fatty acids are important because they help prevent heart disease, high blood pressure, arthritis, and some kinds of cancer. Another group lives only 50 miles away but eats almost entirely grains and vegetables, with very low intake of omega-3's. Both groups eat very low fat diets overall, and both groups have healthy blood lipids and blood pressure. But scientists found that the fish-eaters had lower total cholesterol, lower blood pressure, lower triglycerides, and most dramatically, lower Lp(a)—by 37 percent.

This study doesn't prove whether it's fish or omega-3's that lowered that Lp(a). But along with other emerging news about omega-3's, it adds oomph to what Dr. Castelli has been saying for years: "Eat more fish!" Salmon and white (albacore) tuna are good omega-3 bets.

Broccoli Sprouts: A New Superfood to Fight Cancer

Broccoli has long been touted as a superfood. But now, researchers at Johns Hopkins University in Baltimore have made an unexpected discovery: Broccoli sprouts grown for three days contain from 10 to 100 times more cancer-fighting compounds than mature broccoli does, ounce for ounce. (The compounds—isothiocyanates—help prevent breast and other cancers in animals and probably humans.)

What does that mean to broccoli-haters, and broccoli-lovers, too? You get the power of up to 6½ cups of chopped raw broccoli by eating just ¼ cup of bright green broccoli sprouts. And the taste? Not like broccoli at all. They taste a little like radishes—adding a nice zip to salads and sandwiches.

Since the discovery, broccoli sprouts are cropping up in supermarkets across the country. If your store doesn't have them, ask the store's produce manager about carrying them.

To grow your own, order broccoli sprouting seeds (as opposed to seeds sold for the garden, which may be treated with pesticides) from Johnny's Selected Seeds, 1 Foss Hill Road, Albion, ME 04910. Current seed prices are about $18 per pound or $5.75 per quarter-pound. Prices should fall as the supply catches up with the rocketing demand. One pound has 40 to 48 tablespoons of seeds, and one tablespoon grows 1 to 1½ cups of sprouts. Sprout in a jar (instructions come with the seeds) or order a Bioset sprouter kit for $14.

Is mature broccoli still worth eating? You bet! It has fiber, folate, beta-carotene, and vitamin C at levels far higher than sprouts.

Tomatoes Cut Heart Attack Risk in Half

Tomatoes are red-hot. First came studies showing that people who ate the most tomato products had less prostate and colon cancer. Now, for the first time, we're hearing that tomatoes prevent heart attacks. In Europe, men with the highest tissue levels of lycopene—the compound in tomatoes that may turn out to be the good guy—were only half as likely to suffer heart attacks as men with the lowest levels.

For more lycopene in your life, eat foods such as tomatoes and tomato products, vegetable juice cocktail, watermelon, guava, and grapefruit.

Born to Hate Brussels Sprouts?

Your tastebuds may talk you out of eating healthy. Some people inherit an enhanced sensitivity to certain bitter-tasting chemicals, including those in some foods. Now Adam Drewnowski, Ph.D., and his colleagues at the University of Michigan in Ann Arbor are finding that people with this "supertasting" ability tend to dislike the taste of some phytochemicals—the health-boosting "phytomins" found in vegetables and fruits. One study found that supertasters were much more prone to dislike naringin, a cancer fighter found in grapefruit juice.

To find out if you're a supertaster, Dr. Drewnowski suggests using a cotton swab to paint your tongue with blue food coloring. Check your tongue in a mirror; if it's mostly blue with occasional pink dots, you probably have normal tasting status. If you see many big pink taste buds grouped closely together, the chances are that you're a supertaster.

If so, you may be prone to avoid strong-tasting foods like broccoli, spinach, or kale. But that doesn't mean you're doomed to miss out on the benefits of fruits and vegetables. Carrots, squash, and many deep red and deep orange vegetables contain protective antioxidants, but not the bitter-tasting compounds found in broccoli and its brethren.

Just Incred-Apple

Could an apple a day really keep the doctor away? Yes, a recent study suggests. In Sweden, where rates of kidney cancer are among the world's highest, researchers found that people who ate an apple a day—and just a small apple, at that—had 60 percent less risk of kidney cancer than non-apple-eaters.

Eating more fruit in general was linked to lower risk, too—but the study looked at apples alone because they're so popular in Sweden. In fact, many Swedish families grow their own apple trees in their backyards, says study co-author Alicja Wolk of the University Hospital in Uppsala, Sweden. Orange and dark green vegetables like carrots and kale may also ward off kidney cancer, a previous study found.

Instead of asking Eve, "What's the very best eating apple?" we

Expert	Favorite Apple	What's So Tempting
Tom Douglas (Dahlia's Lounge, Seattle)	Melrose; has a shiny skin, red with yellow background; top growing state: Ohio	Very sweet with a hint of tartness; very firm
Larry Forgione (An American Place, New York City) and Alice Waters (Chez Panisse, Berkeley, California)	Gravenstein; has a yellowish-green skin streaked with red; top growing state: California	Decidedly tart; soft skin with a crisp interior
Jack McDavid (Jack's Firehouse, Philadelphia)	Stayman; has a dull skin, deep purplish red; top growing state: Pennsylvania	Balance of tangy and sweet; lushly juicy and crisp

asked four top gourmets—all owner/chefs of legendary American restaurants. Their favorites? Three full-flavored "specialty" apples (see the chart above) shipped only in small quantities beyond their growing areas. If you find these varieties in a farmers' market or grocery store, pounce. (All can be used for cooking, too.) Or try any locally grown apple; they're often the most flavorful.

Foodstuffs May Unstuff Your Nose

Do you have sinusitis? Try some watermelon. It's full of a substance that may keep your nose unstuffed. A small pilot study done in the Netherlands found that the schnozzes of people with sinusitis were running low on glutathione, an antioxidant compound found in watermelon, grapefruit, oranges, peaches, asparagus, potatoes, and broccoli. The cells that line your respiratory tract need glutathione and other antioxidants to keep free radicals—necessary but dangerous components of your defense system—in check.

According to Irwin Ziment, M.D., respiratory expert and chief of medicine at Olive View–UCLA Medical Center in Los Angeles, there's no proof yet that glutathione-rich foods keep sinusitis away. But adding more fruits and vegetables to your diet certainly won't harm you, he adds, and may be helpful in other ways.

For those who are already stricken with the condition (its hallmarks are a yellow, gray, or green nasal discharge and pain behind your eyes, on the side of your nose, or even in your teeth), you might try carefully sniffing the vapor of hot chicken soup, eating it, or gargling with the broth, suggests Dr. Ziment. The soup contains cysteine, derived from chicken meat, which the body uses to make glutathione.

Ins and "Oats" of Soluble Fiber

Foods in the oatmeal clan have won the right to labels proclaiming that soluble fiber from oats can reduce the risk of heart disease as part of a low-fat diet, thanks to research proving that soluble oat fiber shrinks high cholesterol.

But don't overlook other foods rich in soluble fiber besides oats, especially beans. The new label claim for oats simply echoes a heart-healthy claim that has already been allowed for any food high in soluble fiber.

Prevention advisor James W. Anderson, M.D., professor of medicine and clinical nutrition at the University of Kentucky College of Medicine in Lexington—the doctor who discovered oat bran's powers—recommends aiming for 10 grams of soluble fiber a day. (The Food and Drug Administration says that 3 grams a day is the minimum needed to reduce cholesterol.) Following are a few suggestions of soluble sources to get you started. Unless otherwise noted, all are based on a ½ cup serving.

Kellogg's Bran Buds (⅓ cup)	3.0 g.
Kidney beans	2.8 g.
Lentils	2.0 g.
Sweet potato, cooked	1.8 g.
Quaker Oat Bran, cooked	1.5 g.
Great Northern beans	1.4 g.
1 orange	1.4 g.
Broccoli, cooked	1.2 g.

Pearl barley, cooked	1.2 g.
French-style green beans, cooked	1.1 g.
1 small pear	1.1 g.
100% Bran (⅓ cup)	1 g.
Oatmeal, cooked	1 g.
Quaker Instant Oatmeal (1 packet)	1 g.

Purple Power

A small study suggests that purple grape juice can be as healthy for the heart as red wine. And why not? They're both rich in natural blood-thinning ingredients called flavonoids. At the University of Wisconsin in Madison, people who drank a five-ounce glass of purple grape juice in the morning and evening for a week reduced by 60 percent the tendency of blood to form clots. That's even better than a daily aspirin, which reduced clotting by about 40 percent. (Since clots are the immediate triggers of most heart attacks, anything that prevents them is a major plus.)

Other studies by researcher John Folts, Ph.D., show that one 5-ounce glass of red wine or three 5-ounce cups of tea equal the flavonoid power of 10 ounces of purple grape juice. (Not effective: red or white grape juice, orange juice, grapefruit juice, or purple grape "drink"—as opposed to 100 percent juice.) Will flavonoids replace aspirin? We need more research, says Dr. Folts. If your doctor has prescribed aspirin, don't give it up for grape juice until more information is in.

Update: Selenium versus Cancer

Some of the most prominent cancers today may lose their sting. News has it that the mineral selenium could have potential cancer-fighting powers. Animal trials suggested this in the 1960s, but now the results are in from the first large, well-controlled trial with people. And people taking selenium supplements at the rate of 200 micrograms a day had about half the risk of lung, prostate, and colorectal cancers over the 10 years of the study than did people not taking it.

Better yet, supplement takers had nearly half the risk of dying of any cancer and about a third of the risk of getting any kind of cancer. Ironically, though, the 1,300 people in the study had skin cancer when the study started, and selenium failed to reduce the incidence of new skin cancers. "The skin cancer issue," says Larry C. Clark, Ph.D., lead study author, "is one of the big reasons why we need further research. Also, people in the study were primarily from the southeastern United States, where the soil (and, therefore, the food) is fairly low in selenium." If selenium turns out to be at the heart of the cancer-reduction matter here, that raises the question of whether this reduction would only be seen in those with low blood levels of the mineral. Also, while animal research suggests similar effects would be seen in women, this mostly male study can't resolve that for sure.

Dr. Clark estimates that most Americans get about 100 micrograms of selenium through food, so adding the 200-microgram supplement of organic selenium yeast essentially tripled people's intakes. Just don't go overboard. Toxicity levels have not been clearly established, but some experts warn that there's potential for toxicity at 200 micrograms, while the Environmental Protection Agency considers the safe maximum intake to be a total of around 350 micrograms a day from diet plus supplements. Research hints at serious problems with supplementation over 1,000 micrograms. Selenium often appears in various amounts in multivitamin/mineral tablets; so include that amount in your day's selenium totals if you consider further supplementation.

Veggies with Clout

Ever wonder which vegetables do the most good? One way to judge is to measure total antioxidant power, as a recent study just did. Researchers analyzed 22 commonly eaten veggies, then added up the total antioxidant score (the ability of each vegetable to neutralize disease-causing free radicals).

Mind you, a high antioxidant score isn't the only test of a super-veggie (it doesn't account for fiber or minerals, for example). But the antioxidant score does pinpoint nine veggie All-Stars that belong in your regular lineup because of their superior amounts of total antioxidant power per half-cup helping. Here are the winners, starting with the top scorer.

1. Kale
2. Beets
3. Sweet red peppers
4. Brussels sprouts
5. Broccoli florets
6. Spinach
7. Potatoes
8. Sweet potatoes
9. Corn

Herbal Elixirs

Move Over Aspirin: Seven Herbs to Keep You Out of the Doctor's Office

First, it was an upset stomach as autumn was setting in. Then, a series of headaches in November and that fever last week. And now, a scratchy throat. Before you head to the doctor's office again, stop by the health food store instead. Two of the nation's top herb experts—Prevention advisors Varro E. Tyler, Ph.D., dean emeritus of the Purdue University School of Pharmacy and Pharmacal Sciences and distinguished professor emeritus of pharmacognosy, and Ara DerMarderosian, Ph.D., of the Philadelphia College of Pharmacy and Science—say that there are natural products you can stock at home to help battle the problems that send adults to the doctor most often.

And there are. More than half of these conditions can be soothed, or maybe even prevented, by taking an herb. So if you have a cough to get rid of or hear yourself making the other classic health complaints that follow, consider these expert-recommended herbal remedies.

Licorice

Healers as illustrious as Hippocrates and Pliny the Elder knew of the cough-quelling talents of licorice (*Glycyrrhiza glabra*) back before the Roman Empire. "But there has also been reasonably good research done on its effectiveness lately," Dr. Tyler says. And it looks like ancient doctors knew something about coughs.

How it works: A substance called glycyrrhizin thins what's in your lungs and gives you the "productive" cough that speeds recovery.

How much to take: Dr. Tyler suggests taking licorice in lozenge form because it has a soothing effect on the mucous membranes. One favorite is a licorice-menthol combination called Lakerol (this Scandinavian product is available in the United States in specialty food shops, selected drugstores, and even in IKEA furniture stores). If you're using other licorice lozenges or candy, he says, "make certain that they do, in fact, contain real licorice." Many "licorice" candies manufactured in this country are actually flavored with anise oil. You drink licorice in tea, using a teaspoon or two of licorice-root powder.

Watch out for: Going overboard. "With an excess intake of licorice, your body retains salt and water and begins to lose potassium," Dr. Tyler says, "and that can cause adverse cardiovascular conditions such as an irregular heartbeat."

Echinacea

When you want sore throats and colds to say "uncle" and spare you a trip to the doctor, try taking echinacea (*Echinacea*, various species). Thirty-two stringent studies give strength to the suggestion that this member of the daisy family may prevent a full-blown cold from taking shape.

How it works: Echinacea appears to combat colds in two ways, says Dr. Tyler. One is by activating virus-fighting white blood cells and the other is by stopping cold viruses from spreading out and taking over like kudzu along the highway. (Echinacea may inhibit an enzyme that helps cold viruses canvass your body.)

How much to take: Follow dosage instructions on the bottle. Check the label to make sure that the product is standardized for echinacoside (the active component) and contains *Echinacea purpurea* or *Echinacea angustifolia*. The key is to take it at the first hint of a cold, in tablet or capsule form. The herb is also available in a liquid form, says Dr. Tyler, but he's hesitant to recommend it because the liquids tend not to be standardized, and the echinacoside tends to deteriorate more quickly. Give echinacea one week to exert its cold-fighting effects. While taking it longer won't harm you, Dr. Tyler says, it probably won't do you any good either.

Watch out for: A runny nose and watery eyes. If you're allergic to plants in the daisy family, echinacea will trigger similar reactions.

Chamomile

Mediterranean cultures have been touting the ancient plant chamomile (*Matricaria recutita*) as a cure for stomach ailments for thousands of years. And it turns out that there's a good reason why you should embrace it, too, especially after, say, that pumpkin double-cheesecake.

How it works: A light blue oil within the chamomile plant causes the smooth muscles of the stomach to relax, says Dr. Tyler.

How much to take: As much as you can stomach. If you drink the tea regularly, the therapeutic effect might even add up over time, says Dr. DerMarderosian. Simply put a couple of teaspoonfuls of chamomile leaves in a cup of boiling water, cover, let steep for 15 minutes, and drink up.

Watch out for: An allergic reaction. If you sneeze at ragweed, asters, or chrysanthemums, you're probably going to be allergic to their cousin chamomile as well.

St.-John's-Wort

As a mood booster, St.-John's-wort (*Hypericum perforatum*) has been so effective that it has been approved for the treatment of depression, anxiety, and nervousness by the German equivalent of our Food and Drug Administration. In fact, this herb currently ranks as the number one antidepressant drug—natural or synthetic—prescribed by physicians in Germany today.

The scientific literature confirms that this is no phony. In one 3,000-person study of mildly depressed people, St.-John's-wort improved moods in 80 percent of the people who took it. Even the conservative and highly prestigious *British Medical Journal* found reason to sing the herb's praises.

How it works: St.-John's-wort appears to affect various neurotransmitters on which good spirits are thought to depend, says Dr. Tyler. These include serotonin, epinephrine, and dopamine, the same ones affected by the prescription drug Prozac (*fluoxetine hydrochloride*).

How much to take: Dr. Tyler suggests pouring a cup of boiling water over one to two teaspoons (two to four grams) of St.-John's-wort and letting it steep for 10 minutes before drinking. You should begin to feel more sprightly after about six weeks of drinking one to two cups daily. Whether you buy the herb in the form of tea, powder, oil, liquid, tablets, capsules, or dried leaves, Dr. Tyler recommends buying only those products that are standardized for hypericin, a red pigment in the herb that is associated with quality. Also, follow dosage directions carefully.

Watch out for: An increased sensitivity to sunlight, particularly if you have fair skin. It's true that no cases of hypersensitivity have been reported in people taking normal doses, but light-skinned animals have developed dermatitis and other problems in response to voraciously consuming the herb. Sunscreen is always a good idea.

Feverfew

It can't stop a headache already in progress, but feverfew (*Ianacetum parthenium*), a daisylike cousin of the aster, may help reduce the number and severity of future attacks, especially migraines. That's what British researchers concluded after they reviewed the headache diaries of 59 people who regularly had migraines. They saw that people on feverfew for four months had 24 percent fewer headaches than they did when they weren't taking the herb. (Feverfew gained its original fame in ancient times not just as a headache remedy but as a fever fighter as well—hence its name. This latter talent, however, has yet to be scientifically confirmed.)

How it works: Feverfew's secret weapon is parthenolide, an ingredient that's thought to stop serotonin from flooding into the brain and forcing blood vessels to open wide—and giving you a headache in the process. Feverfew also contains a chemical called tanetin, which may act to reduce inflammation.

How much to take: Dr. Tyler recommends 125 milligrams daily in tablet or capsule form. Make sure that the product has a minimum of 0.2 percent parthenolide (a standard set by the government in Canada). "Feverfew only works if you take it every day," says Dr. Tyler, "and only if you take the recommended dose."

Watch out for: Nonstandardized feverfew sold in the United States, which tends to be inconsistent in quality. Again, be sure to check the label to make sure that you're taking a standardized product.

Herb Alert

When you take any herb, pay attention to your body. If your illness isn't getting better—or if it feels serious to begin with—see your doctor right away. And if you have a serious medical problem or a history of one, talk with your doctor before taking herbs. (And, of course, don't substitute herbs for prescription medications unless your doctor says it's okay.)

Garlic

If you start feeling chest pains, forget herbs and get to the emergency room. But to prevent yourself from getting them in the first place, keep your arteries clean with exercise and a good diet liberally sprinkled with garlic (*Allium sativum*).

A number of both animal and human studies since the early 1980s have shown that this fragrant herb can not only inhibit the formation of clots within the bloodstream but also lower cholesterol and blood pressure levels. "Garlic won't affect a heart condition that's already present," Dr. Tyler says, "but it certainly can be an aid to coronary health in the long term."

How it works: Basically, garlic inhibits the production of cholesterol. Here's how: When a garlic clove is crushed, a substance called alliin meets up with an enzyme called alliinase to form allicin. And that's what scientists believe inhibits an enzyme vital to cholesterol production. Garlic also yields ajoene, which appears to inhibit the formation of blood clots.

How much to take: Take an average dose of four grams (approximately one clove) of fresh garlic daily, says Dr. Tyler. If you don't want to share your garlic breath with other people, "you can buy coated capsules of dried garlic powder that pass through the stomach and release allicin into the small intestine," he says. Expect to take one to four capsules a day, depending on the brand and dosage directions.

Watch out for: Not knowing when to say when. Five or more raw cloves a day may give you heartburn, gas, or related intestinal distress. Some people may even have an allergic reaction. If you're already taking a medication that thins the blood, be sure to check with your doctor about taking large doses of garlic.

Bilberry

During World War II, British Air Force pilots who snacked on bilberry jam noticed that their vision improved when flying at night. Since then, studies with animals and some humans have suggested that concentrated bilberry extract may also help protect against other eye conditions such as degeneration of the macula, the part of the retina that lets us read the fine print on the extract's label. As encouraging as these studies may appear, however, it's going to take more clinical studies before some rigorous scientists are convinced that this berry does everything that it's touted to do.

How it works: The deep purple pigments of the bilberry (*Vaccinium myrtillus*) contain anthocyanins, antioxidants known to help maintain the strength of capillaries. "Some vision problems are caused by minute capillary ruptures," Dr. Tyler says; hence the wisdom of keeping these capillaries as rupture-resistant as possible.

How much to take: Three tablespoons of dried bilberries are all you need. Or, you can boil those three tablespoonfuls in water, strain the liquid, and drink it as a tea. A standardized bilberry extract is available, Dr. Tyler says, 36 percent of which is the active anthocyanins. As for dosage, follow instructions printed on the extract's label, Dr. Tyler says.

Watch out for: Gobbling bilberries in excess. Scientists don't yet know what effect such a binge might have. One more tip: Soften dried bilberries with a bit of water before eating them, or you may chip a tooth.

Best Bets in the Herb Aisle

Herbs, herbs, herbs: St.-John's-wort—a natural antidepressant—on the TV news. Ginkgo—the herb to aid memory—in the newspaper. They're the latest rage. You walk into a health food store to stock up, but the choices are overwhelming.

What is all this stuff? Which kind should you buy? Tablet? Tincture? Capsule?

Which one is better for you: The tablets at 16 cents a pop? Or the capsules for $1.50 each?

> # Five Herbs Not to Waste Your Money On
>
> Why? Because they don't work.
>
> 1. Alfalfa (*Medicago sativa*), for arthritis
> 2. Burdock (*Articum lappa*), as a blood purifier
> 3. Damiana (*Turnera aphrodisiaca*), as an aphrodisiac
> 4. Mexican yam (*Dioscorea composita*), as a progestin-like hormone replacement
> 5. Suma (*Pfaffia paniculata*), as a tonic—it's dangerous

Take heart. Almost everyone is confused and feeling helpless in Herbville. Americans are now spending more than $3 billion a year on herbal products. But the popularity of herbs has grown faster than the speed of American scientists to research them or the Food and Drug Administration (FDA) to regulate them. So how can you get good-value herbs that help, in a form that works?

Simple. Here, the dean of herb experts, *Prevention* advisor Varro E. Tyler, Ph.D., Sc.D., provides the straight scoop on whether or not you should be buying the 10 hottest-selling herbs and which form (capsule, tablet, tincture) works the best.

Here is his advice.

The Top 10: Worth Buying?

1. Echinacea (*Echinacea*, various species): Yes. Echinacea can prevent the common cold. It can also subdue cold symptoms.
2. Garlic (*Allium sativum*): Yes. Garlic lowers cholesterol, thins the blood (which reduces your risk of heart attack and stroke), and fights bacteria like an antibiotic. It may also lower blood pressure and fight stomach, skin, and colon cancers.
3. Ginkgo (*Gingko biloba*): Yes. Ginkgo can aid blood flow to the brain, which perks up memory and concentration. It may also prevent or improve age-related vision loss and other circulatory problems. One recent study even showed that ginkgo helped Alzheimer's patients.

Five Dangerous Herbs

And why.

1. Comfrey (*Symphytum offinale*) for wound healing: it's a carcinogen
2. Coltsfoot (*Tussilago farfara*) as a cough suppressant: ditto
3. Sassafras (*Sassafras officinalis*) as a tonic: again, ditto
4. Germander (*Teucrium chamaedrys*) for weight loss: it causes liver damage
5. Yohimbe (*Pausinystalia yohimbe*) as an aphrodisiac: it increases blood pressure and causes rapid heartbeat (and sometimes nausea and vomiting)

4. Goldenseal (*Hydrastis canadensis*): Maybe. But not for its most popular use, beefing up immunity. It's good on the surface of the skin, not inside the body, where it isn't absorbed. Try it as a topical salve for canker sores or as a mouthwash to soothe a sore throat. One caveat: It's expensive and often adulterated.

5. Saw palmetto (*Serenoa repens*): Yes. Saw palmetto can relieve the symptoms of an enlarged prostate (too many nightly bathroom visits, for one) without the side effects of normal drug treatment, which include impotence and loss of libido.

6. Aloe (*Aloe vera*): Iffy. In its fresh, straight-from-the-plant form, this gel helps heal cuts and burns when spread on the skin. But labels on soap, cream, or lotion rarely tell you how much aloe they contain—mostly very little, says Dr. Tyler. Plus, aloe breaks down with age and doesn't work. So fresh products are essential.

Some people use another part of aloe in capsule or tablet form as a laxative. But it's strong, and Dr. Tyler doesn't recommend it.

7. Ginseng: Yes. Asian (*Panax ginseng*), not Siberian, which actually belongs to a different plant family, is a tonic that tunes up your body and mind and turns up your energy level.

8. Cat's claw (*Uncaria*, various species): Probably not. The Spanish use cat's claw for everything from AIDS to tuberculosis. One

variety of the plant may indeed have immunological powers, but another variety cancels them out. Both types could wind up in the capsule you buy unless you find a product that has no more than 0.02 percent of tetracyclic alkaloids (the plant chemicals that can overpower the other ones). "I'm not sure that there are any products like this available in this country, though," says Dr. Tyler.

9. Astragalus (*Astragalus*, various species): Probably not. Astragalus is popular with practitioners of Ayurveda, an ancient Indian discipline for natural healing. Dr. Tyler says that it has a reputation as an immune stimulant, but there's no substantial scientific evidence to back it up. "Plus, I don't think that there are any standards to check on the reliability of products."

10. Red pepper (*Capsicum*, various species): Yes. The chemical capsaicin that gives hot peppers their heat can also relieve pain. Sold in drugstores as an over-the-counter cream, it is used for such problems as shingles and postoperative mastectomy pain. In capsule form (from health food stores), it can loosen mucous membranes and ease dry coughs from colds.

Up and Coming

Although the 10 herbs above are raking in the most money right now, three more herbs are hot on their heels. Are they worth buying?

1. St.-John's-wort (*Hypericum perforatum*): Yes. This herb is nature's Prozac, Germany's top prescription choice for treating mild depression. It has fewer side effects than synthetic antidepressants. Reports on its benefits are so good, the FDA is studying it for possible approval as a drug (instead of a dietary supplement).

2. Kava kava (*Piper methysticum*): Yes. Kava may be the Xanax of the plant world. Like that drug, it can help you relax or mellow out when you're temporarily suffering from anxiety.

3. Grape seed extract (*Vitis*, various species): Yes. Grape seed extract is a mighty antioxidant. That means it saves cells threatened by free radicals (end products of various oxidation processes in the body) and consequently helps protect us from cancer and heart disease.

Home Remedies

Calm Irritable Bowel with Flaxseed Oil

"I was recently diagnosed with irritable bowel syndrome. My doctor pre-scribed antispasmodic medications, but I wanted to treat my symptoms naturally. I eliminated caffeine from my diet, cut back on sugar and fat, and ate more fruits and vegetables. For added protection, I took flaxseed oil every day. Now this problem is under control—drug-free."
—Jennifer Goldman, Snowhill, Virginia

No one knows what causes irritable bowel syndrome (IBS), one of the most common gastrointestinal disorders. But as Jennifer Goldman dis-covered, the best way to calm an irritable bowel is to modify your diet and lifestyle. Flaxseed oil may be a good place to start: Scientists have found that flaxseed oil is rich in the precursor to an omega-3 fatty acid called EPA (eicosapentaenoic acid), which is valued for its anti-inflammatory effects.

Studies suggest that people with IBS may benefit from adding oils containing omega-3 fatty acids to their diets on a regular basis, says James Scala, Ph.D., nutritionist and author of *Eating Right for a Bad Gut*. Dr. Scala recommends adding two tablespoons of flaxseed oil to your morn-ing cereal every day. (Don't go overboard: There are 14 fat grams per ta-blespoon of oil, so stick to low-fat or nonfat foods as much as possible the rest of the day.)

Silence Hiccups

When I got hiccups as a kid, my mom would give me a spoonful of sugar, which usually worked. Now I offer this folk remedy to my children and friends. Does anyone know how it works?
—Jeff Parker, St. Paul, Minnesota

"No one knows exactly why sugar may help hiccups," says Marla

Tobin, M.D., a family physician in Higginsville, Missouri. "Some doctors speculate that the granules stimulate the vagus nerve, a long nerve in the back of the throat that sends branches to many muscle groups, including those in the diaphragm."

That's why taking a deep breath and holding it for a count of 30 may also work for some. It increases carbon dioxide levels in the blood and apparently decreases the sensitivity of the vagus nerve center in the brain, says Mary Jo Welker, M.D., associate professor of family medicine at Ohio State University in Columbus. "That might be enough to stop the transmission of the hiccups signal."

Another remedy is to close your ears and sip through a straw. Marsha Henderson, R.N., a school nurse in Yorktown Heights, New York, suggests plugging both ears with your fingertips and drinking a glass of water through a straw. "This has worked so well that I even keep straws on hand for it," she says.

A Safe Sleeping Potion

A reader says: *I drink valerian tea occasionally to help me sleep, but a friend told me that it might not be safe. Is valerian tea dangerous?*

Rest easy. The greatest drawback of valerian tea is probably its odor. There is no scientific evidence that the drink is unsafe. Several years ago, a few scientists expressed concern when certain constituents of valerian (*Valeriana officinalis*) known as valepotriates affected the hereditary genes and caused mutations in certain bacteria.

However, valerian tea contains few, if any, valepotriates, which aren't readily absorbed during digestion anyway. In one experiment, only 0.1 percent of the valepotriates originally present in valerian root was found in the tea, and in another study, none could be detected. Commercial preparations (capsules, liquid extracts, and so forth) of valerian usually contain negligible amounts of valepotriates because valepotriates are unstable compounds, decomposing rapidly in storage.

For this reason, the board of German herbal experts, known as Commission E, finds that valerian is a safe and effective sedative and sleep promoter. If you find the tea effective, and its unpleasant odor not too bothersome, there is no reason for concern.

part 2

Boost
Your
Immune
Power

Making Sense of It All

The immune system is the body's natural stronghold against viruses, bacteria, and tumors. The problem is, it weakens over time. And for decades, doctors insisted that there was no way to block this inevitable decline. Thank goodness, new research is suggesting otherwise. There may be preventive actions that we can take after all.

In what has become one of the biggest nutritional breakthroughs, vitamin E is beginning to look like the magic bullet that we've all been waiting for. Taken in levels that are nearly impossible to get through diet, vitamin E heightened the immune response of elderly people. Confirming research is underway.

Meanwhile, Harvard-trained doctor and leader in the burgeoning new field of integrative medicine, Andrew Weil, M.D., offers his sage advice on how we can all help the body heal itself. In an exclusive interview with *Prevention* magazine, Dr. Weil describes all the ways we can keep our immune system humming along with little interference. The body's healing system is what brings us back to health when we get out of balance, he explains. Naturally. Automatically. As long as stress, bad eating habits, or whatever doesn't compromise it. What each of us needs to do is develop an awareness of our body's own healing system, then establish healthy lifestyle habits that encourage this healing system to do what it does naturally. Don't miss reading "Dr. Weil's 10 Ways to Maximize Your Natural Healing Power," beginning on page 52. Follow his advice, and you'll be 10 steps closer to a longer life.

Of course, not every natural remedy touted as an immune booster works. *Prevention* advisor and herb expert Varro E. Tyler, Ph.D., Sc.D., separates the fact from the hype on the popular herb goldenseal (see page 62). He also identifies another herb that does appear to have immune-boosting powers.

All this plus vitamins, minerals, and an exercise prescription that will stir up your immunity and help soften the blow of the common cold.

Positive Action Plans

Rev Up Your Immunity... and Put the Brakes on Aging

At 57, Tina Turner posed for pantyhose ads. Whether or not she's gone under the knife, you can't chalk it all up to plastic surgery.

There's been a remarkable revolution in our ideas about aging. Many Americans are exuding tremendous vitality at a time of life that would have been unimaginable to their grandparents. In fact, most of us hit our strides at an age that would astonish previous generations.

Scientists have also learned that age is not just measured by the calendar. It's now known that the most feared part of aging—that dreaded slide into frailty and dependence—has more to do with biology than chronology. And your biology, in turn, is shaped both by your genetic makeup, which you cannot control, and your lifestyle, which you definitely can.

"You can influence and control your biological age by the way you conduct your life. You can add years to your active life with the right kinds of habits," says Irwin H. Rosenberg, M.D.

Especially your eating habits.

News from the Epicenter of Aging

Dr. Rosenberg should know. He's the director of the Jean Mayer U.S. Department of Agriculture (USDA) Human Nutrition Research Center on Aging (HNRCA) at Tufts University in Medford, Massachusetts. The center—one of six research institutions sponsored by the USDA—is the only one devoted exclusively to studying the links between nutrition and aging.

Since research on aging began in earnest in the 1970s, some of the most significant findings in the field have come out of here. Granted, they haven't discovered Ponce de Leon's dream, a wellspring of eternal youth. But they have come to an important conclusion: All of our various body parts and biological processes don't age in the same way. Rejuvenation then comes from drinking from not one Fountain of Youth, in a sense, but from many fountains.

"There are general laws of aging that influence all tissues, but there are also highly specific functional changes that go on in different organ systems with age," says Dr. Rosenberg. "And they may be quite different from one organ to another. Aging of the eyes may be quite different from the aging of the skin, which is in turn quite different from the aging of the lungs."

Dr. Rosenberg turned that insight into a book, *Biomarkers: The 10 Keys to Prolonging Vitality*, which he cowrote with William Evans, Ph.D., who is now at the University of Arkansas in Little Rock. The 10 measurements determine how old you really feel, and they can all be altered by proper diet and exercise. Now, seven years later, Dr. Rosenberg has more good news. The latest research seems to be uncovering two important new biomarkers: 1) our brains, and 2) our immune systems. Eating the right foods may help us keep our minds clear, quick, and sharp and help fight off disease for a long, long time.

Brain Power Forever

Headlines brought news of a previously unknown risk factor for heart disease: homocysteine. This amino acid, when present in the blood at elevated levels, is suspected of damaging artery linings, making them more susceptible to atherosclerosis. Because of that, homocysteine may be a trigger that causes 10 to 15 percent of all heart attacks.

What you may not have read is this: High homocysteine levels may affect your brain as well as your heart.

It's been known for some time that arteries occluded by cholesterol can lead to strokes, and that strokes, large or small, result in cell damage that affects normal brain function. (They also affect speech, gait, and memory, depending on where in the brain they occur.) It's also known that the B vitamins play an important role in nervous system function. When the human brain sputters along without adequate amounts of B vitamins, disorders like depression and dementia may be the unfortunate result.

But are there even subtler forms of nutritional deficiencies that may not result in such outward, obvious symptoms? Does nutrition influence cognitive function in otherwise healthy people? Those are the key questions, and scientists are beginning to find some answers.

The first piece of the puzzle was picked up in the early 1990s, when a team of HNRCA researchers, led by Dr. Rosenberg, looked at the 1,041 surviving elderly people from the famous Framingham Heart Study. The scientists found an association between high homocysteine levels and gunked-up carotids—the arteries on either side of your neck that carry oxygen to the brain. So it's entirely possible that the brain cells of people with high homocysteine levels are not getting an ample supply of nutrients.

Then researchers Karen Riggs, Ph.D., and Avron Spiro III, Ph.D., added another finding. When they gave 70 elderly veterans a battery of cognitive tests, they saw an association between low levels of vitamin B_{12} and folate and high levels of homocysteine in the blood and poor performance on a test called spatial copying, in which the men were asked to copy geometric figures like circles and cubes. "The subjects with the highest homocysteine concentrations performed, on average, like patients with mild Alzheimer's disease," they wrote.

The next step in the research will be to conduct magnetic resonance imaging (MRI) scans on people with high homocysteine levels and poor cognitive test scores to see whether they suffer from blobs of dead brain cells. "We know there's something happening in the brain, but we don't know what the homocysteine is actually doing," says Dr. Riggs. "We'll have to find out what's happening at the level of the brain cell to tie together these two findings."

The science here may be confusing, but at least it boils down to some easy nutrition advice. Homocysteine levels are kept in check by adequate amounts of vitamins B_6, and B_{12} and folate in your daily diet. Aim for the Daily Values: 2 milligrams of B_6, 0.4 milligram of folate, and 6 micrograms of B_{12}. To get what you need, make foods rich in these vitamins a part of your healthy diet and consider taking a multivitamin to make up for any shortfall.

"Cognition is a particularly complex area," says Dr. Riggs about her chosen field. But it can yield tantalizing evidence—like the findings contained in a chart taped to her office door. At first glance, the chart, obscurely titled "Survival by Quartile of Gs," means nothing. All it shows is three downward-trending lines. But to Dr. Riggs, it means plenty: The three lines represent the death rates of men who took part in a veterans' study back in the 1960s. It shows that the men who were the fastest at

10 Ways to Maximize Your Natural Healing Power

Harvard-trained physician and integrated medicine leader Andrew Weil, M.D., recommends the following 10 tips to help you make the coming year your Year of Optimum Health.

1. Develop greater awareness of your healing system. Think about your own healing experiences. Focus your thoughts on how your body was able to heal itself, with or without outside treatment.

2. Switch to olive oil. Buy a bottle of extra-virgin olive oil and use it as the main source of fat in your diet. Cut down as much as possible on your use of saturated fat, polyunsaturated vegetable oils (except for expeller-pressed canola, which is fine for you), and trans fatty acids (partially hydrogenated fats).

3. Eat more fruits and vegetables. Because researchers continue to identify more and more protective compounds in fruits and vegetables, eat the real thing. Don't be misled into believing that you can get all the benefits of fresh fruits and vegetables by taking a supplement that just contains the isolated compounds.

4. Develop your breathing. Sit in a comfortable position with your back straight, your eyes slightly closed, and your clothes comfortably loosened. Focus your attention on your breathing and follow the contours of your breathing—inhalation and exhalation—noting, if you can, the points at which one phase changes into the other. Do this for five minutes a day. This is a basic form of meditation to harmonize body, mind, and spirit. Turning your attention to breath moves you naturally toward relaxation and meditation.

taking various perceptual and motor speed tests (such as plugging pegs into holes) are the most likely to be alive today: 88 percent of them, in fact. Whereas, of the men who were in the slowest fourth of the group 29 years ago, only 52 percent are alive today.

"Whatever was affecting their brain function was starting to show up 30 years ago," Dr. Riggs observes. Could it be that degenerative diseases sneak up on your mental acuity long before they show up in a doc-

5. Walk every day. You cannot enjoy optimum health if you are sedentary. Walk at least 45 minutes a day, five days a week.

6. Spend time in nature. Connecting with nature is a simple form of meditation that takes us out of our routines and keeps us from being too focused on our thoughts and emotions.

7. Take supplements that fit your lifestyle and health history. For most people, I recommend a daily routine of the following in these specific amounts.

   • 1,000 to 2,000 milligrams of vitamin C two to three times a day
   • 400 to 800 international units of vitamin E
   • 200 micrograms of selenium
   • B complex with at least 400 micrograms of folic acid and no more than 100 milligrams of B_6
   • ½ regular aspirin (162 milligrams) with food, unless you are allergic or have a bleeding ulcer

8. Cut down your intake of toxins. Drink only bottled water or install a water purification system in your home. Eat organic and local produce whenever possible.

9. Learn about tonics. Tonics are natural products that increase the efficiency of the healing system and help neutralize harmful influences. Some of the most powerful tonics include garlic and ginger (eat more of them), green tea (drink it instead of coffee), and ginseng (it's good for people who lack energy or vitality).

10. Seek out positive practitioners. Be sure that your health care practitioner has faith in your ability to heal. Do not regularly see a doctor who thinks that you cannot get better; the beliefs of health care practitioners strongly influence your healing power.

tor's diagnosis of heart disease or high blood pressure? That's a lifetime of scientific inquiry right there.

Super Immunity Plan

One of 16 laboratories at the HNRCA is the Nutritional Immunology Laboratory. This is where Simin Nibkin Meydani, Ph.D., investigates the role of nutrients in boosting the immune system, the body's natural line of defense against viruses, bacteria, and tumors. The problem is, the whole system gets out of whack with age. It actually becomes deregulated, says Dr. Meydani. When that happens, we have less resistance to disease.

Like most scientists, Dr. Meydani has spent years finding out what doesn't work. A recent study of black currant seed oil, for instance, found no immune-boosting effect. But she is excited about her current work on a more commonly known nutrient: vitamin E.

Vitamin E is necessary to the body, although cases of deficiency are rare in Western cultures because we get it in our high-fat diets. Nonetheless, for decades, some people have consumed supplemental amounts in the form of vitamin E capsules, based on their own hunches rather than on any clinical scientific evidence, which was virtually nonexistent.

Then, in the 1980s, scientists realized the key role played by vitamin E as an antioxidant. It soaks up free radicals, which are produced by the interaction of oxygen and fats in the body. In doing so, it protects the cells of the immune system from damage. Now that the mechanism is understood, says Dr. Meydani, "it makes sense that vitamin E would enhance the immune system." (It's also possible that vitamin E protects artery walls from getting gunked up with cholesterol.)

Dr. Meydani had two major studies published in 1997. In one study of 88 elderly people, those who took vitamin E for four months showed greater immune-system response, as measured by antibodies in the blood, than those who received only a placebo. (The optimum level was 200 international units per day; many times above what it is possible to get from food.) A second study, in which old mice were given megadoses of vitamin E, showed that the daily supplement offered some protection against an influenza virus. Notably, this study was the first in which "a higher than adequate intake of a nutrient has demonstrated a beneficial effect on influenza in animals."

So Dr. Meydani appears to be one study away from saying conclusively that vitamin E supplements—beyond what you'd get from a healthy diet—do indeed enhance an older person's resistance to infectious disease. And that one study is under way. It involves 634 residents of nursing homes in the Boston area. It will test the effects of vitamin E supplementation on flu infections. Final results are three to four years away.

Secrets of Age-Stopping

"Nutrition science moves forward by little steps that add together to develop a picture," says Dr. Rosenberg. Here are some components of the big picture as they have begun to emerge.

Exercise. Starting at age 40, most women lose nearly one-third of a pound of muscle a year, replacing it with fat. By age 80, they have only one-third of the muscle tissue that they had at 40. But this slide is not inevitable: Exercise has been shown to restore muscle mass, strength, and balance, even among people in their nineties. One study of nursing-home residents with a mean age of 87 showed that three 45-minute sessions per week with muscle-building resistance machinery worked wonders. Not only did muscle strength double and stair-climbing speed increase by 30 percent, but a few of the participants were able to throw away their walkers and canes.

Exercise prevents a whole host of age-related problems from developing, including frailty and osteoporosis. "It's extraordinary what exercise can do—it's the unrecognized Fountain of Youth," says Miriam E. Nelson, Ph.D., associate chief of the physiology laboratory at the HNRCA and author of *Strong Women Stay Slim* and the national bestseller *Strong Women Stay Young.*

Calcium. According to at least one study, elderly people who eat a healthy diet and take calcium and vitamin D supplements will cut their risks of bone fractures in half. Vitamin D helps the body absorb calcium. Bone loss is a major problem among postmenopausal women with low calcium intakes, and the greatest rate of decline occurs in the first five years after menopause. A National Academy of Sciences panel recently recommended that people over age 50 get 1,200 milligrams of calcium a day—the equivalent of four 8-ounce glasses of fat-free milk.

B vitamins and folate. A diet rich in vitamins B_6 and B_{12} and folate may reduce the risk of heart attack and stroke by reducing homocysteine levels. And although many women think those causes of death are "a guy thing," they are in fact the leading causes of death among postmenopausal women.

Vitamin C. The most common age-related eye problem—cataracts—can be delayed or avoided by getting enough vitamin C. A study of 247 women (mean age 62) shows that women who took vitamin C supplements for 10 years or longer lowered their risks of getting

Good, but Not Guaranteed

What puts the chill on a cold virus? Researchers have been stalking the answer to that question for decades—and now they have a few more findings to report.

Drink C and see. Once you have a cold, vitamin C can help reduce the duration and severity of your symptoms. That's what one Finnish researcher found when he analyzed and compared the results of numerous vitamin C studies. "Researchers are just beginning to understand how it affects our immune systems," says Barbara Levine, R.D., Ph.D., associate professor of nutrition in medicine at Cornell University Medical School in New York City. "Many of the studies that have been done have not been well-controlled or well-done." Plus, when it comes to actually preventing colds, vitamin C may fall short for most of us. Some Finnish research suggests that C's cold-stopping power is limited to just a few groups of people, such as strenuous exercisers or people whose vitamin C intakes are already low.

Make more friends. The more varied and abundant your social ties, the safer you may be from a cold, suggests a study done at Carnegie Mellon University in Pittsburgh. Of 276 adults exposed to cold viruses, those with the widest variety of social contacts also had the lowest cold risk—half that of their counterparts who were the least social. It may be that a broad spectrum of friends (provided they cover their sneezes) may help us deal more effectively with stresses that lower immunity.

Tip a few. In a study of 400 men and women by Carnegie Mellon and the Medical Research Council in Salisbury, England, people who averaged one to two alcoholic drinks a day were 16 percent less likely to get sick when exposed to a cold virus than a control group who never raised a glass. The study's author, Sheldon Cohen, Ph.D., speculates that alcohol may alter a cold virus's ability to reproduce or that alcohol may act as an anti-inflammatory that inhibits cold symptoms. No one is suggesting that you belly up to the bar just to prevent a cold, but if you're headed that way, you may also head off a cold.

Caution: While alcohol may be beneficial when it comes to colds, other research suggests that even as little as one drink a day may increase a woman's risk of breast cancer.

cataracts by greater than 75 percent. Simply sticking to a diet rich in vita-min C may achieve the same results; another HNRCA study indicates that eye tissues are saturated with vitamin C at intakes between 150 and 250 milligrams per day.

Beta-carotene. Foods rich in beta-carotene appear to have a protec-tive effect against all cancers. But beta-carotene supplements are not rec-ommended. In dosages of more than 30 milligrams per day, they seem to have little benefit and may even be harmful. In one study, smokers con-suming 30 milligrams of beta-carotene saw an increase in lung cancer.

Cholesterol. Research in the center's Lipid Metabolism Laboratory has demonstrated that women who are past menopause and men who are over age 50 with moderately high cholesterol can make a difference in their levels by switching to a low-saturated fat, low-cholesterol diet. The average reduction of 10 to 15 percent in low-density lipoprotein (LDL) levels is enough, in some cases, to move a person's cholesterol level out of the danger zone without drug therapy. The center is one of the few studying the effects of low-saturated fat, low-cholesterol diets in older individuals. Previously, most data had been collected from college-age males.

Burning calories. Studies of body energy balance provided no evi-dence to support the conventional belief that some people have a God-given ability to burn off more calories than other people, and that's why they're so thin. People become overweight because of an imbalance be-tween the food they consume and the energy they burn—and a remark-ably small imbalance of only 2 percent results in 80 extra pounds after a decade. As we age, the excess pounds are harder to lose.

Ironically, although nutrition knowledge has been expanding, it was largely ignored by a nation relentlessly focused on a single nutrition topic: fat. "We were fat-obsessed in the 1980s," says Dr. Rosenberg. "The single message that got out was about fat, and in the end, that was a disservice to the public. People came to think of nutrition education as what they needed to know about fat, when, in fact, other nutrition messages were also important."

The obsession with fat obscures the HNRCA's overall message—that exercise and a healthy diet can empower your old age. "It has been remarkable and very exciting to be here all this time," says Dr. Nelson, who began working at the center in 1983. Back then, she recalls, few believed that proper nutrition and exercise could make a big difference in people's lives. But the difference is truly profound. And Dr. Nelson looks back and marvels, "We never thought it would turn out to be as profound a difference as it is."

Five Ways to Stop Your Next Cold

With cold viruses lurking on everything from doorknobs to dollar bills, avoiding a cold can seem like dodging snowflakes in a blizzard. But the chances of keeping your nose clear in the year ahead may actually not be so bad. Here are five ways that scientists have found to stop your next cold, or at least soften its blow.

1. Buy yourself flowers. Strange as it may sound, a purple member of the daisy family may head off your next cold. Thirty-two clinical trials indicate that the herb echinacea boosts the immune system. "It activates the specialized white blood cells that help destroy invading organisms such as cold viruses," says herb expert and *Prevention* advisor Varro E. Tyler, Ph.D., Sc.D. "It also inhibits an enzyme that causes the invading cold virus to pass from cell to cell."

Echinacea appears to be most effective when taken at the first signs of a cold. No harm has been associated with more extended use, but no benefits have been observed either. Dr. Tyler recommends buying the tablets or capsules (available in most health food stores) and following the dosage directions carefully. Check the label to make sure that the preparation you buy comes from either *Echinacea angustifolia* or *Echinacea purpurea* and that the mixture has been standardized.

2. Exercise, don't agonize. Forget "no pain, no gain." Moderate, not strenuous, exercise is the hero when it comes to cold-stopping powers. "Every time you take a brisk walk, it increases the circulation of immune cells through your body," says David C. Nieman, Dr.P.H., professor of health and exercise science at Appalachian State University in Boone, North Carolina. That increase jacks up the chances that immune cells will meet up with and combat the cold virus. In three different studies, Dr. Nieman and his team of researchers found that women who walked fast enough to moderately boost their heart rate (30 to 45 minutes, five days a week) had half the illness rate of women who remained sedentary.

And more is not better. Exercise intensely for more than an hour, and stress hormones kick in. "Those can suppress the immune system," says Dr. Nieman. "After a marathon, for example, a runner's risk of illness is six times greater than normal."

Don't think that one walk a month can bestow these protective powers. "A brisk walk gives a nice little boost to the immune system," says Dr. Nieman, "but only with near-daily activity."

3. Zinc fast. It might sound unsavory, but taken in lozenge form, zinc appears to have some pretty impressive powers against colds. In a study at the Cleveland Clinic, for example, 50 people with colds who sucked on lozenges packed with 13.3 milligrams of zinc every two hours kissed their symptoms good-bye in almost half the time of their placebo-popping counterparts.

Still, the study's author, Michael Macknin, M.D., is reluctant to say that his research is definitive. "It's exciting information, but until any medical treatment has been studied many times, you can't be confident that it definitely works," he says. Of seven other studies, three reported similar benefits and four did not. Dr. Macknin suspects that different formulations may have affected the outcomes.

How zinc works is also uncertain, says Dr. Macknin, but he offers several theories: One is that zinc prevents the cold virus from hooking onto the respiratory tract and causing an infection. Another theory is that zinc may block the growth of the virus's outer coat, stunting its ability to multiply. Zinc may stimulate production of the body's virus-fighting natural substance, interferon, or it may shore up cell membranes, making them less vulnerable to viral infection in the first place.

Zinc lozenges (the most common brand name is Cold-Eeze) are available in most drug, grocery, and health food stores. Another option is a peach/apricot-flavored lozenge containing 23 milligrams of zinc, which you can find in some health food stores. Zinc lozenges have some side effects: About 80 percent of the patients said that they had an unpleasant aftertaste, and 20 percent were nauseated. To combat nausea, Dr. Macknin recommends sucking the lozenges on a full stomach.

Caution: Only use zinc lozenges when you have a cold, not on a regular basis. Too much zinc can actually impair immune system functioning.

4. Make a habit of hand washing. Washing your hands as often as possible is the first line of defense against colds, advises cold expert George L. Kirkpatrick, M.D., clinical associate professor of emergency medicine at the University of South Alabama in Mobile.

But we're not talking about just any kind of hand washing. According to one study, the proper hand-washing technique is equally important (no quick rinses allowed here). A group of teachers and school-age children who were taught to wash their hands thoroughly and properly wound up getting fewer colds during a 10-week peak cold–season period than did a similar group who washed their hands in the usual hurried manner.

"Washing properly means wetting your hands with water and lathering up with an antibacterial soap," says Dr. Kirkpatrick. "Rub all the surfaces of both hands together, including the insides of your fingers, for at least two minutes. Then go up the wrist, and then pick under your fingernails to clean out the debris." Dr. Kirkpatrick washes his hands approximately every five minutes when doing patient care in the emergency room, but unless you're a doctor, every five minutes probably doesn't fit into your schedule. Aim for a scrub before or after hand contact and especially before and after you eat, change diapers, or go to the bathroom.

5. Keep your distance. It's a maxim that most of us learned at Mom's knee, but it seems that Mom was right (again): The basic way to avoid a cold is to avoid people with colds. That was the verdict reached in a study by the University of Helsinki in Finland and the National Institute of Public Health in Oslo, Norway. The study found, not surprisingly, that your risk of catching a cold rises in proportion to the extent of the company you keep. Makes sense. Each time a cold victim sneezes or speaks, he sends volleys of viral water droplets through the air, as far as 30 feet. Even a well-intended handshake can pass along a cold virus. "If your immune system is strong, you may not get a cold," says Dr. Kirkpatrick. "But you're now carrying the virus. Touch your child, she gets a cold, and then you wonder where she got it."

So do you vow never to leave the house? Of course not. We need to be with people. In fact, at least one recent study suggests that having a wide variety of friends can help reduce the number of colds you get. Still, you can reduce your chances of sharing their germs or spreading yours. Make it a house rule that all coughs and sneezes get well-buried in a tissue that then goes directly into the trash. "It's probably worthwhile to wipe off countertops and tables with disinfectant immediately before everyone congregates for meals, since the germs will repopulate the surfaces in about 30 minutes," says Dr. Kirkpatrick. "And don't share toothbrushes, glasses, or teacups." Other smarts: Shop when crowds are smallest. And postpone your child's play date until Billy is over his cold.

Why haven't flu shots been mentioned? Flu shots attack only the viruses that cause influenza, a separate illness with some coldlike symptoms, like runny nose and coughs, but primarily characterized by a head-to-toe body ache.

Sage Advice

Your Ticket to a Longer Life

We work hard for our health. We take the stairs instead of the elevator. We jump up and down in aerobics classes until we sweat more than a mailman on Spiegel catalog delivery day. And we like it. But wouldn't it be nice if there were at least one easy way to extend our life expectancies?

Actually, there are several ways, including shows, concerts, museum exhibits, and even ball games. This good news comes from Sweden, where a large study found that people who frequently attended cultural events tended to live longer than those who attended them less often.

How can sitting through Beethoven's Fifth do you good? One explanation is "vicarious emotional arousal," according to study author Lars Olav Bygren, M.D., of Sweden's Umea University. "Emotion influences the body's systems that combat disease," he explains. So when a concert or play wows you, it may be spurring your immune system or other disease-fighting resources to be all that they can be.

This doesn't mean you should trade in your running shoes for tickets to *Don Giovanni*. But do consider heading to the theater when you're done at the gym. It could be your ticket to a longer life.

Safeguard Your Zinc

The zinc in a woman's entire body weighs less than one green pea, but it's vital for a strong immune system. Now a study at Tufts University in Medford, Massachusetts suggests that women who take in recommended levels of calcium (1,000 to 1,500 milligrams a day) might wind up with lower zinc levels. What to do? Don't curtail your calcium. Until we understand this interaction better, Tufts mineral expert Richard Wood, Ph.D., says that it makes sense to take a multi-supplement with 15 milligrams of zinc—100 percent of the Daily Value—but no more. It's okay to take multis and calcium supplements together.

Herbal Elixir

Goldenseal: Can This Herb Boost Immunity?

Herb expert and Prevention *advisor Varro Tyler, Ph.D., Sc.D., separates the fact from the hype.*

Learning the truth about an herb as popular as goldenseal may feel a little like finding out that there is no Santa Claus. Still, in a field where misinformation abounds, it's better to know the truth.

The herb consists of the underground parts (rhizome and roots) of a small American forest plant, *Hydrastis canadensis.* Its common name, goldenseal, derives from the herb's intense golden yellow color. Native Americans used the plant for war paint, clothes dye, and to treat skin conditions and sore eyes.

Today, goldenseal is the third–best-selling herb in the United States. It is widely touted as an immune booster, for which it is often combined with another herb, echinacea. The combination product is used mainly to

How to Use Goldenseal

Goldenseal won't keep you disease-free, but if it's a natural anti-septic that you want, it'll do the trick. For mouth sores or sore throat, steep 1 teaspoon in a cup of hot water for 15 minutes. Use the tea as a mouthwash, swishing it in your mouth every three to four hours.

If you have traveler's diarrhea, take ½ to 1 gram in capsule form, three times daily.

ease symptoms of the common cold. If the mixture works, however, it's due to the echinacea, not the goldenseal. The results of more than 25 controlled clinical trials give good reason to believe in echinacea's immune-boosting ability. Goldenseal, on the other hand, lacks scientific support, and what scientists do know about this herb withers any chance of its boosting immunity. Lots of hype, little research.

There has been little scientific study of goldenseal's usefulness. Even in Europe, well-known for its study and use of herbs, goldenseal has not been investigated. Nor is it used frequently. The few studies that have been carried out are flawed by the fact that the alkaloids that are the active constituents in goldenseal were usually injected into animals. Since goldenseal is taken orally, that's how the studies need to be conducted. Otherwise, the results are very different.

When taken orally, berberine and hydrastine, the main active alkaloids in goldenseal, are not absorbed well from the digestive tract—that is, they do not get into the bloodstream. If an herb or drug doesn't get into the bloodstream, it can't work systemically (throughout the body). Goldenseal cannot pump up the immune system if it can't get into the bloodstream.

That's not to say goldenseal is good for nothing. The alkaloids of goldenseal, especially berberine, have significant antiseptic activity against a fairly wide range of bacteria. This activity makes goldenseal a potentially effective treatment for such local infections as mouth sores, throat conditions, and traveler's diarrhea.

At one time, berberine was widely used in this country as an antiseptic agent in various eyedrops. It is still so used in Europe. With such limited usefulness, it's surprising that goldenseal is so popular. But stories about other benefits of this so-called golden herb started growing. Myths fuel popularity. About 20 years ago, the herb acquired a considerable reputation on the West Coast for masking drug tests. Claims were made that consumption of goldenseal "purified" the urine of heroin addicts, thereby masking the results of typical urinalysis tests. This myth was soon extended to include tests for cocaine and marijuana, as well.

It is believed that all the hoopla is based on the misreading of an episode in *Stringtown on the Pike*, a novel written in 1900 by pharmaceutical researcher John Uri Lloyd. But the fact is that goldenseal is more likely to cause false-positives than to prevent detection of illicit drugs. Still, no amount of debunking seemed to discourage would-be users, and the popularity of goldenseal climbed to new heights. The results are a limited, high-priced (about $50 a pound) supply of goldenseal. Most of the domestic supply is wildcrafted—collected from wild-growing plants because it is hard to cultivate. It takes three to four years for the rhizome and roots to reach a harvestable age. Consequently, goldenseal is frequently adulterated with the underground parts of other species containing yellow-colored alkaloids. When the plant material has been finely powdered or otherwise processed, such adulteration is difficult to detect, and probably renders the product less effective.

Goldenseal thus remains an interesting example of a little-researched, relatively unimportant herb that through hearsay and hype has acquired an undeserved reputation.

part 3

The Rewards of Simple Living

Making Sense of It All

You've picked your closets clean. You've trimmed your magazine subscriptions to what you have time to read, and not one page more. With tricks for doing just about everything faster, from mowing the lawn to shuffling the kids off to school, you tear through your calendar like that Looney Tunes creation known as the Tasmanian Devil. So why, at the end of each day, do you feel like someone has dropped an anvil on your head?

Simplicity is the essence of healthy living. By paring down to life's essentials, you carve out more time for healthy pursuits, like taking a daily walk, having fun with your kids, or just doing nothing (for a change). And, as a bonus, when life is simplified, you feel less hassled, less burdened. You can breathe easier. You feel less stressed.

So where do you begin?

Check out "Real-Life Solutions for Simple Living." These everyday tips come from real people who simplified their own lives (out of true necessity). Learn their secrets and find your own peace in the process.

Then turn to page 72 for some "Simple Tactics to Shrug Off Stress." Here's where you'll discover how to reap the rewards of a more simplified lifestyle. Discover some of the mental tricks and physical techniques that can help you stay healthy—from meditation and afternoon tea to on-the-job advice to help tackle difficult projects.

Not surprisingly, people are discovering ever more secrets to escape the health-depleting effects of stress. In "Three Minutes to Total Relaxation" on page 82, you'll find a simple meditation routine that virtually eliminates the stress-producing "chatter of the mind." Or turn to page 83 to discover a potent herb with anxiety-reducing and muscle-relaxing effects. Even dancing and breathing have their own stress-relieving rewards.

Positive Action Plans

Real-Life Solutions for Simple Living

Simplifying our lives is all well and good, but too often, we rush to save time only to turn around and fill it with another task. The tips that follow are designed not just to cut corners or speed a process along but to streamline your life as well. These tips will take the hassle out without your having to set aside a Saturday or two in which to do it.

To lend things a personal touch, we tracked down real-life authorities on simplicity. These folks aren't your run-of-the-mill, jargon-spouting experts. And they're not the Oprahs and the Madonnas who have entire staffs to simplify their lives for them. These are real people who really are doing it all: Among them are a mother of quintuplets, the president of a major university, and a rat-race dropout sailing around the world solo. Each of them adds a unique twist to the word *simplify*.

So, before you decide that your life is muddled beyond hope, read on and see for yourself. The answer is simple.

Fire the paper boy. He's probably saving for college. But most major newspapers (and not a few smaller ones) are on the Web, and going there is more efficient all around.

- News online is usually fresher than the version on your doorstep.
- In all but a handful of cases, online newspapers are free (no bills to pay).
- There's no need to stop delivery when you're on vacation.
- There's no need to drive a month's worth of papers to the recycling center.
- And, as a bonus, you don't waste time scrubbing ink off your hands.

Pass the bills. Want to save paper, stamps, and licking time? You can automatically pay your bills—and always on-time—if you sign up for automatic bill-paying at your bank. Contact yours to find out how.

Lose your answering machine. Bid farewell to call waiting and junk those tiny cassettes that fill up your drawers and seem to jam on all but the most banal of messages. How? Residential voice mail. You can take messages whether you're on the other line or away from home or simply not in the mood to chat. Plus, you can send messages without having to talk to a real live person. Ask your phone company for details.

Buy a notebook and keep it handy. Jotting down shopping lists and plot lines for your Great American Novel is a good idea; just don't do it on whatever scrap happens to be lying around. ("Hey, I was using that napkin!") Merge such imperatives onto one master list. And make it big so it's easy to find.

Phone ahead. Right before you leave for your appointment with the dentist, optometrist, or whatever "-ist" you're due to see, call to make sure that the good doctor is running on schedule. You have better things to do with your time than sit around listening to Muzak.

Make them come to you. Hunt around for a dry cleaner that picks up and delivers. If you're a regular, you just might merit special treatment.

Hire a haggler. Shopping for a new car can feel like a boxing match. So get someone to step into the ring for you. Write to CarSource at P.O. Box 513, Kentfield, CA 94914, with the make, model, and options that you're looking for in your new car, then kick up your heels. CarSource contacts dealerships within a 60- to 90-mile radius of your home to find the very best deal, then sends you in to inspect your new vehicle and hand over the check. That's it. The fee runs from $275 to $675, depending on the price of the car, but CarSource guarantees savings from $1,000 to $12,000.

Wash without water. Once you've bought your new car, you'll want to keep it nice and shiny. But rather than spending every Saturday in the driveway (or blowing a stack of quarters at the local car wash), use the Kozak Auto Dry Wash. It's a 15- by 36-inch rag designed to wipe away dust and light dirt. It won't scratch your vehicle's finish, and it's good for up to 50 cleanings. It's available for $9.95 (plus shipping) by writing to Kozak at P.O. Box 910, Batavia, NY 14021.

Stamp out stress. If you have a credit card, cross the post office off your to-do list and pick up the phone. The U.S. Postal Service will deliver stamps to your mailbox within approximately five business days. Be sure to ask for their Stamp 24 menu when ordering. This menu changes every few months, but recently, a minimum order of 60 32-cent

Think Survival

Ever wish so hard for a dream that you finally went out and just did it? Even if it meant sacrificing comforts that so many of us think we can't do without? After six years of wishing and a lot of planning, Karen Thorndike did exactly that. The 54-year-old quit wishing and did it, selling her house in Seattle to sail around the world. Solo.

Preparing for her trip, Thorndike couldn't afford to indulge in espresso machines and curling irons (she had to cram her whole life into a 36-foot boat). By necessity, her life was streamlined. "I emphasized the items that help me survive," she says. "Food, water makers, clothing." Even if you never venture past the mall, it's a useful frame of mind to adopt.

stamps costs $22.20, including shipping. Check with your local Post Office for details.

Get to know your librarian. Even if your local library doesn't have a cappuccino bar, it still beats out the local Book-Mart. Why? Look no further than the teetering pile of "must-reads" on your nightstand. Buy a book, and its presence is a nagging reminder of unfinished business until you've read every last chapter.

And then it sticks around for 10 more years after that. Borrow one, and you can simply dump it in the night-return box and be free of it.

Do your work—and no one else's. The fastest way to add to your workload is to gain a reputation as a know-it-all. "A man I know liked to be thought of as the resident expert, so whenever there was a problem, he was the guy to turn to," says C. Steven Manley, Ph.D., a psychologist in Dallas. "He ended up working until midnight just to finish his own work."

Close the book. "Read any good books lately?" Good luck trying to escape a dinner party without hearing that one. Thing is, staying hip to the latest bestsellers can be draining, to say the least. Instead, simply read the reviews (the *New York Times Book Review* is a sure bet). They dish up enough highlights to see you through any casual conversation and provide ready-made commentary to boot. Before long, you'll be spouting phrases like "spellbinding narrative" without even trying.

How It's Done

Want some real-life inspiration to help you simplify? The princi-ples can be summed up in four words: delegate, focus, reflect, and re-examine. Here are some people who took these principles to heart—and what happened.

Delegate. Becky Mangus isn't interested in preserving the bound-aries of home and work. For one thing, it loses some meaning when your office is at home. For another, as she illustrates, habits learned at work often help keep her home life humming.

Mangus, who runs her own graphics-design company in Ellicott City, Maryland, recalls a turning point. She says that a few years ago, she collapsed from sleep deprivation. "So I was forced to slow down and sim-plify," she says. For instance, she realized that while she charged $50 an hour for her time, a messenger service charged $16 an hour. The decision was a no-brainer. Soon, she was doling out responsibilities left and right.

"My husband and children all help out. When there's work to do, we all pitch in." And, Mangus says, she has learned when to simply let things go. "My priorities don't include a 100 percent immaculate house," she says. "And that's okay with me. I made that decision."

Focus. Just try to find a book on simplification that doesn't quote Henry David Thoreau. The nineteenth-century writer's exhortation to "simplify, simplify, simplify" is catchy, no doubt about it. But what's be-hind it?

"It's not as simple as going into the woods and shutting your ears," says Joel Myerson, Ph.D., professor of American literature at the Univer-sity of South Carolina at Columbia and editor of *The Cambridge Compan-ion to Henry David Thoreau.* "Thoreau really focused on what's important. He thought of what he didn't like, articulated why he didn't like it, and proposed an alternative." In other words, stop and think: Is this really worth hours of my life?

"Whenever I'm offered an administration job, I say no," Dr. Myer-son says. "I don't think the payback is worth the time that goes into it."

The key word here is *think.* For instance, consider Dr. Myerson's basement. "Henry would be disappointed in me," he admits. "I'm a book collector." At first blush, it looks like clutter, an affront to the very idea of simplicity. But look again: "There aren't great collections of New Eng-land literature here in the South," says Dr. Myerson. "And it's easier to collect books in my basement than to waste time in Boston doing research."

Cluttered basement versus jetting to Boston several times a year? In the end, the clutter wins hands-down. Gee, maybe Henry would approve, after all.

Reflect. Father Leo O'Donovan seems perfectly suited to teach simplification. After all, as a Jesuit priest, Father O'Donovan gives his salary directly to the Jesuit community, has no real possessions, and quotes Saint Ignatius of Loyola from memory.

On the other hand, Father O'Donovan also happens to be the hands-on president of Georgetown University in Washington, D.C. "Today? At 4:00, the chancellor of Germany is coming over, and then tonight we're having a dinner for a cardinal from Rome. My life is simple," he says, pausing. "And complex."

It's complex in the sense that it's impossible to lead a major university without a date book crammed to overflowing; simple, in that through it all, Father O'Donovan remains cool and in control. Even his voice is soothing.

"The biggest challenge is prioritizing and trying to give your best to the most important things," he says. "Being a Jesuit helps. We have a spirituality that encourages us to be as simple as possible. We're not saying that you have to take a vow of poverty; there's an easier way to unclutter your life."

In a word: reflection. "Give yourself time to reflect," he says. "In a society as fast-paced as ours, that's hard. And many people find it uncomfortable just to sit and be with themselves. But taking that time every day really helps."

Skeptical? Just try it, "today," Father O'Donovan urges. See if a bit of reflection doesn't lend your life a bit more clarity. "I think that even if you don't have a religious tradition, it's very healthy and very simplifying."

Take music, he says. "The other night, though I didn't have the time, I stopped and put on Mozart's twenty-seventh piano concerto." He pauses again. "I was very happy for the 25 minutes that it lasted."

Reexamine. Last summer, Amy and Eric Guttensohn got a crash course in simplification. Once before, the Montgomery, Alabama, couple had tried in-vitro fertilization, and failed. But the second attempt paid off in a big way. Each of the four embryos that the doctors implanted grew, and one split into twins, just for good measure. On August 8, 1996,

Amy gave birth to quintuplets Mason, Tanner, Hunter, Parker, and Taylor, and learned to simplify. Fast.

"I was never an organized person," says Amy, 29. "But when the boys arrived, we had to sit down and reexamine everything." Here's her new philosophy.

Bulk up. "Buying in bulk helps," she says. "Stock up as much as you can to cut down on trips to the store." (This works for toothpaste and canned soup as well as it does for diapers.)

Know when to fold 'em. Or, more important, know when not to, Amy says. "Laundry that doesn't need folding, I don't fold," she says. "I know mothers who fold cloth diapers over and over and over. I throw mine in a pile."

Stow away. If your kitchen has more gadgets than a department store showroom, maybe it's time to do some pruning. Amy says that this was her first step toward a simpler house. "Anything that we weren't using every day, we stowed in the attic," she says. "Our ceilings are ready to collapse under all the weight."

Simple Tactics to Shrug Off Stress

We all love the sweet things in life, but when the pace becomes too hectic, we discover to our distress that we can't pack it all in. And then along come the not-so-sweet surprises—a stack of unpaid bills, a bad review at work, or news that an ailing parent has taken a turn for the worse. The stress inducers are all around us.

What do we do?

As strange as it may seem, the key is to stop fighting it.

"Stress hits when you feel like you're not in control," says Paul J. Rosch, M.D., clinical professor of medicine and psychiatry at New York Medical College in Valhalla and president of the American Institute of Stress in Yonkers, New York.

To master stress, then, you need to distinguish between the things that you can do something about and the things that you can't. Once you learn to change your mindset, you can get a reprieve from many of stress's body- and soul-sapping consequences.

Basic Steps to Counter Stress

This simple tactic works wonders, but unfortunately, it can't eliminate stress from your life. Nothing can. That's why it's so important to create a sense of tranquillity and control in your life to help ensure that stress doesn't get the upper hand.

Actually, all it takes are some simple steps.

First, build stress breaks into your schedule. "You need to spend time relaxing every single day," says Herbert Benson, M.D., president of the Mind/Body Medical Institute and director of behavioral medicine at Beth Israel Deaconess Medical Center, both affiliated with Harvard Medical School, and associate professor of medicine at the medical school. "In fact, my recommendation is a 10- to 20-minute session twice a day." The stress breaks written into your appointment book should be inscribed in ink.

Second, customize your stress-management routine. The more time you devote to things that you enjoy—bird-watching, doing jigsaw puzzles, sitting down to an hour of needlework after dinner—the less time you waste stewing about things that you can't control.

A rule of thumb is to do something positive and do it regularly. "That's the key to managing stress successfully," says Allen J. Elkin, Ph.D., director of the Stress Management and Counseling Center in New York City.

Fast-Acting Mental Stress Busters

You don't have to become a Zen master to master relaxation techniques—some can defuse stress within minutes with these everyday tips.

Do the dishes. You can transform any task, even washing the dishes, into a calming ritual, using a mental technique called mindfulness, writes Jon Kabat-Zinn, Ph.D., in his book *Full Catastrophe Living*. As described by Dr. Kabat-Zinn, director of the University of Massachusetts Stress Reduction Clinic in Amherst, and one of the forerunners in bringing "mindfulness meditation" into the mainstream, mindfulness is the ability to focus intensely on what you are doing.

Concentrate on each plate, glass, and fork as you wash it. Notice how your fingers, hands, and body move as you hold, scrub, and rinse. Think of nothing but those dishes, as though you could wash them with the intensity of your focus. Learning to live in the moment has many benefits, writes Dr. Kabat-Zinn. "Cultivating mindfulness can lead to the discovery of deep realms of relaxation, calmness, and insight within yourself.

See your way clear to easy land. Who has time for a vacation? You do, when you use a mental technique called visualization.

Close your eyes and think of a peaceful place you've been. Inhale deeply through your nose and exhale through your mouth as you mentally relive a perfect afternoon at the lake or in the woods. Chances are, you'll feel more relaxed in less than a minute, says Michael A. Tarrant, Ph.D., professor of forest recreation at the University of Georgia in Athens, who has studied the psycho-physiological effects of imagining past nature experiences.

Dr. Tarrant and his colleagues found that after people recalled these experiences, they reported feeling more relaxed. "Some people's mental states improved after only one minute of visualizing," he says.

Repeat yourself. Relaxation is a skill that can be developed to help with stress, says Jon Seskevich, R.N., who teaches stress reduction techniques to seriously ill people and their families at Duke University Medical Center in Chapel Hill, North Carolina. Repeating a phrase silently to oneself over and over also has a calming effect. When the mind wanders, simply return again and again to the phrase.

Try repeating "The Lord is my shepherd," inhaling on "Lord" and exhaling on "is my shepherd." Or try "easy does it," breathing in on "easy" and exhaling on "does it," says Seskevich. As you concentrate on the phrase and your breathing, your stress will begin to fade.

Get some R&R. Rapid relaxation, that is. This 30-second technique "is a simple way to let go of tension—to become sort of like a limp rag," says Dr. Elkin.

It's simple to do. When you feel yourself getting stressed, Dr. Elkin says, touch your thumb to any finger on the same hand and press them together, hard. As you do this, take a deep breath through your nose. Hold that breath for five seconds or so. Then, part your lips slightly and exhale. Release your fingers as you imagine a wave of relaxation spreading from the top of your head to the tips of your toes.

Make like Pavlov's dogs. Take a few minutes to pinpoint which everyday occurrences regularly make you tense. For most people, the stress inducers are things like sitting down to pay bills, answering the phone at work, or trying to zoom through intersections before the yellow light turns red. Mentally link these stress signals to a relaxation exercise.

"Hearing your office phone ring might be your cue to take five seconds to stretch or breathe deeply before you pick up," suggests Dr. Elkin. "Or an adhesive dot stuck to your steering wheel reminds you to do a mental exercise like rapid relaxation when you hit a string of red lights or a traffic jam. These prompts can really help take the edge off your stress."

Burst some bubbles. When nothing else works, bubble wrap comes in mighty handy. Popping these sealed air capsules reduces stress, according to a study conducted by Kathleen Dillon, Ph.D., a psychologist and professor at Western New England College in Springfield, Massachusetts.

It's a throwback to the classic worry bead, a smooth stone that the ancient Greeks carried with them and rubbed between their fingers to release tension. "Playing with the poppers seems to have the same effect as a lot of nervous habits, but there are no side effects," says Dr. Dillon. "It's a lot better than smoking cigarettes."

Stress-Management Exercises

Stress-management exercises are like situps: The more often you do them, the more you benefit. But to get really good at them, you need to practice. Here are some stress blasters worth learning.

Breathe with your bellows. Most people breathe using the muscles in their chests. But chest breathing actually perpetuates stress and makes your heart and lungs work up to 50 percent harder, according to Phil Nuernberger, Ph.D., author of *The Quest for Personal Power: Transforming Stress into Strength*. Dr. Nuernberger notes that many mental disciplines, including yoga, teach another breathing method to relax the body and focus the mind.

Breathe using your diaphragm, the dome-shaped muscle under your lungs, advises Dr. Nuernberger. Using that muscle like a big expanding bellows, you actually pull air into the blood-rich lower lobes of the lungs. This allows the lungs to work more efficiently than they do during chest breathing.

Make your ratio two to one. While breathing with your diaphragm, try two-to-one breathing to relieve stress. If you exhale twice as long as you inhale, these drawn-out exhalations help relax and quiet the body, according to Dr. Nuernberger.

Learn to meditate. Meditation, which triggers the relaxation response, is a proven stress reducer that's also good for your heart. It lowers blood pressure and cholesterol levels and may even help people with heart problems live longer, healthier lives. Researchers from the State University of New York at Buffalo and the Maharishi University of Management in Iowa taught a small group of men with heart disease how to meditate. After eight months, these men were able to exercise 14 percent longer and 12 percent harder than a group of nonmeditators.

Make a motion to lose stress. In China, people in middle and old age can be seen in public parks practicing tai chi. A gentle kind of martial art, tai chi is a form of "moving meditation" that tones the muscles while it calms the mind.

Research has shown that even gentle exercise, like tai chi, is the best antidote for stress. Even a short walk helps burn off stress hormones lingering in the blood and release endorphins, hormones that give you a feeling of well-being.

"Walking or other moderate exercise produces a holistic pattern of change—what I call general body arousal," says Robert Thayer, Ph.D., professor of psychology at California State University of Long Beach. "Your heart rate and metabolism increase. The tension in your muscles goes down. And there are changes in hormones and in brain neurotransmitters, which have a significant effect on thinking and mood."

5- to 15-Minute Moves

When it comes to beating stress with exercise, every move counts—even tiny ones. These 5- to 15-minute moves are proven stress busters.

Give yourself some rope. Just a few minutes of jumping rope can help reduce stress, says Daniel M. Landers, Ph.D., a researcher at the Arizona State University Exercise and Sports Research Institute in Tempe. Since it's an aerobic activity, jumping rope gets your heart pumping, moving stress hormones out of your system. You can even jump rope at work. If you have an office with a solid door, put on your sneakers and skip away tension in privacy.

Stretch out your neck. Taking a minute to stretch will loosen the muscles in your neck and shoulders, which tend to knot up when you spend hours staring at a computer monitor or sitting at a desk. Here are two ways, recommended by Dr. Landers, to help stretch your neck muscles.

1. Take a deep breath, drawing your shoulders up toward your ears. As you exhale, bring your shoulders down and back.

2. Take a deep breath and, as you exhale, turn your head as far to one side as you can. Hold for 10 to 15 seconds, breathing evenly. Repeat, turning your head to the other side with the next exhalation.

Take your brain for a stroll. Forget speed-walking around the mall. Instead, take a meditation walk—a slow, comfortable stroll that research has shown can reduce anxiety as well as a brisk walk.

In a meditation walk, pay attention to your footsteps, counting "one, two, one, two." If you find your thoughts drifting, think, "Oh, well," and return to counting your footsteps. A group of people who practiced this technique over a 16-week period reported feeling less anxious and more positive about themselves.

Home, Stress-Free Home

If coming home from work isn't any more soothing than actually being at work, your home may not be the haven that it could be.

"Most people don't realize how profoundly their home environment affects them," says Carol Venolia, an architect and the author of *Healing Environments*. And she's not just talking about decor. "Sometimes they don't think about how things like light, sound, and air quality can affect them," observes Venolia.

One of the simplest ways to make your home a more soothing place is to welcome in natural light. Spending too much time in artificial light can disrupt your body's daily rhythms, which can cause stress and fatigue, research shows. Natural light is not only—well—more natural, it also conveys real information about time and weather, and that's information your body needs to maintain its natural rhythms.

To get more natural light every day, you might need to change your sleeping arrangements so that your bedroom gets morning sun. Or rearrange your kitchen so that the breakfast nook is against a sunny window. While it might seem odd at first to convert your study into your bedroom, you may also feel more energetic once you're getting the natural light that your body needs.

In addition to getting more light in your life, there are other things you can do to stress-proof your home. Some take just minutes to accomplish. Try these quick home improvements.

Take off your shoes. In Japan, people exchange their shoes for slippers as soon as they get home. Buy a cushy pair of slippers and keep them right beside your front door. This simple shoe-swapping ritual can help you make the transition between the stress "out there" and the serenity of home.

Brew a cup of tea. "There are few hours in life more agreeable than the hour dedicated to the ceremony known as afternoon tea," wrote Henry James in *Portrait of a Lady*. So unpack grandmother's china tea set, brew a cup of tea (decaffeinated or herbal), and spend a few minutes savoring its flavor, aroma, and soothing steaminess. "Little touches like this are extremely important," says Venolia.

Broaden the spectrum. They may be energy efficient, but fluorescent lights are not what you'd call soothing. "Most fluorescent lights are the old-fashioned kind that hum and flicker and make your skin look sickly," says Venolia. But she points out that newer fluorescent lighting is now available that provides illumination much closer to natural light. Full-spectrum fluorescent lights, as they're called, actually mimic the full-spectrum light of the midday sun.

Light a single candle. You don't have to reserve candlelight for romantic dinners. "This kind of warm, low-level light is soothing because it's primal," says Venolia. "It still touches a place in us. You get a similar feeling from this kind of light that you do from watching the sun set."

Spotlight for atmosphere. Keep general lighting levels lower. But if you want to read or do needlework, use a small, brighter task light, like a clip-on lamp, Venolia suggests.

Pick up the scent of serenity. Research shows that pleasant aromas encourage relaxation. In studies at the Royal Berkshire and Battle Hospitals in Reading, England, researchers found that critically ill people treated to the scent of lavender oil felt more positive and less anxious. Lavender, apparently, seems to increase the brain's production of alpha waves, a tangible measurement of relaxation. To reap those soothing benefits, look for naturally scented soaps, oil, and candles that can lend a benign, soothing fragrance to your home environment.

Clean out the sniffle makers. Constantly being sick can be stressful, says Venolia, and that's how you may feel if you're allergic to something in your house. Before Venolia found out that she was allergic to mold and took measures to control it, she recalls having constant colds and respiratory problems.

After Venolia's doctor determined that she was allergic to mold, she cleaned out hidden mold sources in the closets, bathroom, and bedding. The problems downsized, and stress diminished.

If allergies are making you tense and exhausted, be sure to get tested by an allergist. If you do turn out to have an allergy, you may end up cleaning more often. But it's a small price to pay to release some stress, reclaim your former vigor, and make your home a more welcoming place.

Bring the outdoors in. Think of how peaceful you feel when you listen to the patter of raindrops on leaves or see a mother duck drift across a pond with her ducklings. "Feeling connected to living things reduces stress," says Alan M. Beck, Sc.D., a professor of ecology at Purdue University in West Lafayette, Indiana.

One way to connect with nature is by bringing plants into your home. "I have two or three bookshelves that are filled just with plants," says Venolia. "I believe that seeing plants is healthy, and caring for them certainly feels good."

Noise-proof your home. If there's street noise outside your window, it can filter through, adding to your stress more than you realize. Investing in double- or triple-pane windows, weather stripping, and thermal insulation can reduce outside noise, says Venolia. You can also reduce reverberation inside your house with fabric wall coverings, cushy furniture, and carpeting. "All of these absorb noise," she notes.

Go to some land Down Under. Some grade-school teachers set aside one corner of their classrooms as a sort of stress-free zone, says Venolia. "Kids who need time out can retreat to this corner. It might have a pile of soft pillows to lie on, books to look at, and tapes of nature sounds to listen to. There might even be a little bowl of potpourri." This corner is called Australia or Antarctica—a land far, far away from the stresses of the classroom.

To create mini-Antarctica for yourself, set up one room—or even one corner of a room—as your private place to sip a cup of tea, suggests Venolia. Use that retreat to practice stress-reduction exercises or perhaps just browse through a favorite magazine. "It may give you some much-needed peace," she says.

Put Work Stress in Your Out Box

The hours are long and the pay is lousy. Your boss doesn't listen to you. Nobody appreciates what you do. The copy machine is always jammed, and your voice-mail light is always blinking. In other words, you have no control.

Yes, you do, says Jeanie Marshall, an empowerment consultant and founder of Marshall House, a Santa Monica, California, company that trains people and organizations to be more effective. To beat stress at work, says Marshall, you have to move from feeling beleaguered to feeling empowered.

"Empowerment isn't power that somebody 'gives' you," says Marshall. "You already have it." But the first step is knowing what you can change and what you can't. Being aware of what's beyond your control actually makes you feel less helpless. You'll also become more efficient and productive, says Marshall, because you won't waste time trying to fix the unfixable.

While empowerment may seem like an imposing challenge, small changes can count for a lot. Here are some instant actions that can help define your area of control—and also help take the stress out of work.

Ask the right question. When you feel powerless in some conflict with a co-worker, or you're feeling helpless in the face of a looming deadline, ask yourself how you can get some control over the situation. If it's a co-worker issue, the answer might be to talk over the problem with your colleague. If it's a deadline that's giving you the jitters, why not break the project into easy-to-handle parts and focus on one part at a time.

What's the benefit of approaching problems this way? "A sense of control," says Marshall.

Make a "priority card." Write your priorities on an index card, keep the card in your desk, and glance at it frequently. "It can be a helpful tool in the first few weeks and months if you forget what your priorities are," says Marshall. But at some point, the card will become irrelevant and you won't need to remind yourself any more. "Then you know that you've internalized your priorities," she says.

Have a five-minute vent. Ranting to a trusted co-worker about a botched project definitely reduces stress. The problem is, most of us don't know when to quit. "Vent for five minutes, then be done with it and move on," says Marshall. That way, venting becomes a conscious decision instead of an unconscious reaction that fuels stress.

Make a different kind of list. Many time-management experts advise making a to-do list and checking off each item as you do it. But this technique doesn't work for everyone, says Marshall. "A lot of people find list-making very frustrating because they still don't get things done."

Another approach is to write down what you *have* accomplished, suggests Marshall. By allowing you to feel good about your accomplishments, you will find that such a list pushes you to move on to doing other things so that you can add them to the "done" list rather than the "to-do" list. "I suggest that people try this when they feel overwhelmed with things to do," says Marshall. "They usually come alive because they realize that they really have accomplished a lot."

Just say it. Learning to say no—to committees, projects, even requests for help—is one of the simplest ways to stay calm on the job, says Marshall. Of course, you don't want to refuse every task, every colleague, and certainly not your boss. But if you're not sure when to say no, check your priority card. If the task doesn't match one of your priorities, nix it if you can.

Don't give your all. It's important to work at a capacity that replenishes us rather than depletes us, advises Marshall. "If we work at 80 to 95 percent capacity on a regular basis, we tend to feel exhilarated at the end of a day rather than exhausted. And when we are required to give more than 100 percent, we find that the extra reserves are available."

Make excellence good enough. Perfectionists often work harder and less effectively because they can't let go of one project to attend to others. Also, they may procrastinate, which adds to their stress. "When priority one bumps up against priority two, which bumps up against priority three, we need to decide when—and what—we're willing to let go," says Marshall. If you go for excellence rather than perfection, there may be a few bugs in a project. But it gets done. If you're trying to eliminate every last flaw, a single project can take forever.

Do many things, focus on one. "Working on one project while worrying about the other that just hit your desk not only makes you tense, it makes you less effective," Marshall says. So give your full attention to one thing at a time, no matter how busy you are, she advises.

Don't sweat the mess. Many people think that if their offices are neat and their files alphabetized, they'll automatically become more productive. Again, the self-inflicted pressure to get organized may actually work against you, especially if you're the creative type. So if your desk and filing system seem disorganized but you know where everything is, "let go of feeling guilty about the mess," says Marshall.

Sage Advice

Three Minutes to Total Relaxation

On the road to simplification, even relaxation rituals crave paring down. After all, a 20-minute meditation twice a day takes too much effort for "simple living." Fortunately, the road from "in over your head" to inner peace just got shorter with these simple techniques from the book *The Three Minute Meditator* by David Harp and Nina Feldman, Ph.D.

In fact, says Harp, you probably do some form of meditation already, even if you don't call it that. "Whenever you keep your attention so strongly focused on something that no other thoughts intrude, that's a form of meditation. Hang gliding is a meditation for some, harmonica playing for others." The point is focusing your awareness on just one thing. The result is that the usual chatter of the mind (stress–producing chatter) is stilled.

Here are two of Harp's best three-minute routes to total relaxation via simple meditation.

1. Count your breaths. Simply count mentally as you exhale each breath: "Inhale . . . one, inhale . . . two, inhale . . . three, inhale . . . four," then begin again with "inhale . . . one." Strive to not lose your count and try not to alter or regularize your breathing in any way. Try to feel the physical sensation of each breath, both inhalation and exhalation, as it passes through your nose or mouth.

If you find yourself thinking about anything except the feel of your breath and the number of that breath, return to focus on the sensation of breathing and on the number of that breath. If you are not absolutely sure what number breath you're on, begin again with "inhale . . . one." No judging, no "I blew the count" thoughts, just back to "Inhale . . . one."

The beauty of this meditation is that, once learned, you can do it anywhere. Try it while waiting in line or at the Laundromat (no one can even tell that you're doing anything).

2. Count your heartbeats. Every second, your heart beats at least once. So counting or labeling each beat is an amazingly powerful attention focuser, even if you do it for only one minute or less. Locate your pulse in your wrist with a few fingers. Count each beat or pulse to 4, like you've done with your breath.

Herbal Elixir

Nature's Stress Buster

Simplify your life and live stress-free. Do you wish that it were that simple? In truth, all the 'simplify your life' tactics in the world can't banish stress entirely. But don't despair. Regular exercise and natural relaxers like deep breathing and three-minute meditations should keep everyday stress at bay. And when, occasionally, a period of extra stress overwhelms you, it's nice to know that Mother Nature stocks a soother in her medicine chest. Here's one of the best, described by herb expert and Prevention *advisor Varro E. Tyler, Ph.D., Sc.D.*

Kava kava (*Piper methysticum*) is a relatively new (to the United States) herbal product that can enhance relaxation, especially welcome when you're feeling temporarily bowled over by life or particularly anxious in the face of a predictable stressor, like a fear of airplane travel, for instance.

For hundreds of years, kava kava has been used as the key component of a Pacific island nectar used in religious and social rituals. Islanders grate the underground stem of the kava plant, mix it with water, and strain it. Drinking the resulting beverage creates a feeling of pleasant relaxation.

Mellow Maker

I'm enthusiastic about kava's usefulness for people today. The results of five well-designed, well-conducted German studies from this decade involving more than 400 people were all positive. For example, in 1995, 100 people with anxiety and stress (resulting from family or job-related situations and even menopause) were given 210 milligrams of kava's active compounds (kavapyrones) a day. After eight weeks, the people taking the kava were clearly improved in comparison with those receiving a placebo.

The German Commission E, which is responsible for evaluating the safety and efficacy of botanical medicines (and is recognized as the world's leading authority on herbs), gave kava its stamp of approval in 1990. They found the herb beneficial for relieving nervous anxiety, stress, and restlessness.

Kava's anxiety-easing and muscle-relaxing effects are due to some 15 different chemical compounds known as pyrones, collectively named kavapyrones or kavalactones. These act on the central nervous system and generally produce noticeable results within about ½ hour to 2 hours.

How Much Calm Can You Take?

With an herb as potent as this one, there is understandable concern about possible side effects. Observations of more than 4,000 patients consuming 105 milligrams of kavapyrones daily for seven weeks noted 61 cases (1.5 percent) of undesired effects, which included mostly mild and reversible stomach upsets or allergic skin reactions. A four-week study of 3,000 patients taking a higher dose (240 milligrams daily) produced a slightly greater incidence (2.3 percent) of similar side effects. Commission E's recommended daily dosage is 60 to 120 milligrams of kavapyrones (or kavalactones), enough to be effective but with minimal side effects.

Long-term consumption of kava above those levels may result in a yellow discoloration of the skin, nails, and hair as well as allergic skin reactions, visual disturbances, and difficulty in maintaining balance. For this reason, Commission E recommends that it be taken for no longer than three months without medical advice. Kava should not be used if you are pregnant, nursing, or suffering from depression. To ensure safety, it's best to consult your physician prior to using the herb, especially if you have been using any psychoactive drug.

If you're interested in trying kava, look for a standardized product containing kavapyrones or kavalactones. Often, those products are standardized to contain 30 percent kavalactones. (That means that in a 150-milligram capsule, there are about 50 milligrams of kavalactones.) So to stay within the recommended dosage, you could take two of these capsules a day. It's wise to start with the lowest dose to gauge its effects.

Like antihistamines, kava may impair your ability to drive or operate machinery. You would want to observe your reactions carefully and follow the same precautions you would when taking any substance that might impair your performance. Kava should be reserved for particularly stressful times in life, not used for everyday anxieties. If you should feel that you need to use it longer, see your doctor.

User Discretion Advised

Strangely enough, interest in kava started to grow just as the Food and Drug Administration began to express concerns about the safety of another psychoactive herb, ephedra. Although both substances affect the mind and behavior, their specific effects on the central nervous system are very different: Ephedra is a stimulant; kava is a depressant.

Kava is a potent, effective medicine, and therefore, also subject to abuse. If the American herbal industry markets it in a responsible manner, and we use it appropriately, we will have a very useful herb added to our therapeutic resources. If not, kava products are certain to become subjected to rigid controls to limit abuse.

Home Remedy

Dance Away Stress

———

At the end of a long workday, I need something simple to help me switch into home gear. The nearest gym is an hour away, and I have a husband and three kids waiting for me to come home. Just when I thought I was out of luck, I heard about movement meditation. This form of dance has renewed my sense of self and gives me enough energy to last until bedtime.

—Blythe Kanis, Davis, West Virginia

Based on the ancient concepts of traditional Chinese medicine and yoga, movement meditation combines breathing and gentle, flowing movements to create a meditative state.

"It allows people to draw in chi energy from the earth, which many healers such as acupuncturists regard as the essential life force," says Eileen F. Oster, a meditation instructor from Bayside, New York. Chi (pronounced "chee") is energy that moves along meridians, or paths, throughout the body. It is an essential concept in Traditional Chinese Medicine.

Here's how Oster recommends that you practice movement meditation.

Center and concentrate. Take several deep, cleansing breaths. Then, move into a relaxed squatting stance with your knees slightly bent and your hips and pelvis loose. Center yourself by visualizing your feet connected to the soil. Visualize the center of the earth, from which we draw our energy, says Oster.

Focus your awareness. Gently move your body in an undulating, snakelike, swaying motion. See yourself as a flower opening up or as an animal moving through the brush. Dance, if you like.

Use music to focus your attention on the movement and on the vibration. Allow yourself to get lost in the sense of movement and the beauty of your body as it moves. Feel the areas of your body that are tight and let the movement loosen them.

Healing Moves

Breathe Easy

One surefire clue that stress has you in its grip is short, shallow breathing. You can tell in an instant. Place one hand on your chest, another on your abdomen, and feel the movement. If your chest is expanding but your belly isn't, you're not handling stress as well as you could. By breathing deeply, so that your abdomen expands like a balloon, you can automatically calm both mind and body. Take a few deep breaths right now and feel the difference. Then, to help maintain a deep breathing pat-

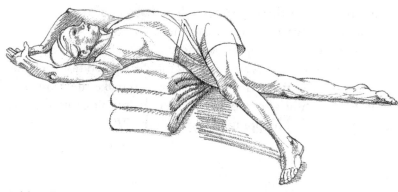

Stretching Back

Fold three or four firm blankets into long rectangles. The blankets should be soft but not too squishy when you lie back on them. Stack them 8 to 16 inches high. Lie sideways over the blankets with your waist well-supported. Lie exactly on your side, not rolled onto the front or back of your body. Center your waist so that both your shoulder and hip are suspended. Stretch your arms gently overhead. Move your top leg forward and your bottom leg backward equally from the center line. Stay for 30 to 60 seconds or longer, taking full breaths. To switch sides, bend your knees and use your hands to press up to sitting.

Note: If your back hurts, lower the height of the blankets. You should be comfortable but still feel the stretch.

For extra stretch, grasp the wrist of the arm on top with the hand from below, and gently pull.

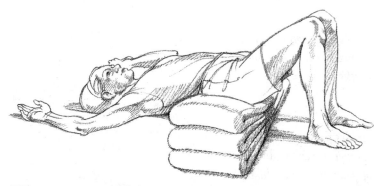

When coming out of the stretch, roll onto your back, resting your pelvis on the blankets and your shoulders on the floor. Stay for a few soft breaths. Then, moving your body in the direction of your head, slide off the blankets until your hips rest on the floor. Breathe for a few moments before rolling to one side and pushing up.

tern, simply practice these easy stretches that target the oft-neglected muscles of the ribcage and sides of the chest.

These deceptively simple-looking stretches also can provide a profound effect, calming nerves and melting muscle tension from achy necks, shoulders, and backs in no time at all. Why not make the most of a few moments of downtime after work or dinner by dropping into these relaxing soothers instead of plopping in front of the TV?

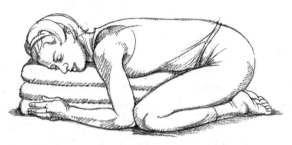

Child's Pose

Fold three blankets into rectangular shapes long enough to support your torso and head fully when you bend forward. Stack them on top of each other. Bring your big toes together and stretch your buttocks back toward your heels. Rest the full weight of your stomach and chest on the blankets. Place your arms on the floor near your head. Stay in this position with your eyes closed, breathing gently, for about 5 minutes. Halfway through, turn your head to the other side. Eventually, work up to 10 minutes.

If your knees feel strained, put a blanket between your heels and your buttocks.

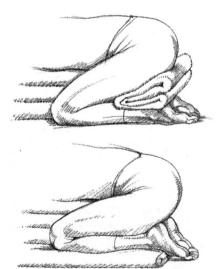

If your ankles feel stiff, place a folded blanket under the full length of your shins. Let the tops of your feet hang off the end. Keep adding height until you're comfortable, raising the height of the chest support accordingly.

part

4

Natural
Weight
Control

Making Sense of It All

The secret to losing weight is really no secret at all. The bottom line is that you have to burn more calories than you consume. Simple. So why is it so darn difficult?

For maximum calorie burn, it is now known that you don't have to exercise longer or harder—just smarter.

New research has proven that strength training is the key to stoking your metabolism so it burns white-hot all day long. In as little as two 20-minute sessions per week, you can amass significant muscle stores, which makes losing weight faster and easier. That's because the more lean muscle you have, the more calories your body burns over the course of the day—whether or not you're physically active.

Of course, burning body fat requires aerobic activity, like brisk walking or jogging. But by strength training, your aerobic workouts will become more efficient. With more muscle behind your workouts, you'll burn fat faster. That means less time on the treadmill. Whew!

Feel flabby in all the wrong places? Well, you've heard over and over again that spot reducing doesn't work. It's true; you can't preferentially burn fat from a given trouble spot. But good news, a combination of fat-burning aerobics and resistance training that "spot tones" specific muscles can give you the physique you want even if you can't lose weight. Learn exactly how right here.

Whatever your personal weight-loss stumbling block, these chapters have the latest, most effective, action plan for you. After all, it's not just what you eat, it's how you eat. It's not just how much you exercise, it's what kind of exercise you do—and whether you enjoy it. It's not just about your body, it's about your head. And it's not just about body weight, it's about body fat and muscle.

Here, the best new research, the most knowledgeable experts, and the most successful "personal weight managers" help you fine-tune your weight-loss program for success. Losing never felt better.

Positive Action Plans

Take Off the First Five Pounds Fast

Slow and steady is the way to go if you want to lose weight permanently. But you can shift into high gear to get started and see healthy results in just one month.

Doubt it? Take a look at Melanie Griffith, Goldie Hawn, Kurt Russell, Pierce Brosnan, and supermodel Vendela. When these stars need to get control of their bodies, they turn to personal trainer Greg Isaacs to help them shed extra pounds, shrink their waistlines, and firm their arms and legs. When the cameras roll, they're tight and toned. But contrary to what you may think, Isaacs' clients are not spending endless hours in the gym, subsisting on celery sticks, or having their chefs spend hours in the kitchen. His philosophy is "get your diet, get your exercise program, and get a life."

With Isaacs' expertise, we have created a diet and exercise program that will take off those extra pounds fast. And you'll spend minimal time thinking about it. Everything is outlined in the easy-to-follow steps below, and by the end of the month, you'll be slipping into your "skinny" jeans, no problem.

Easy Does It

The program consists of daily meal plans and exercise prescriptions that are time-efficient. It's the quality of both the workouts and the diet, not the quantity, that's important. "Less is actually more," Isaacs says, when it comes to workouts. But you have to commit to the diet as well. "If you're not going to pay attention nutritionally, and you're going to work out, you're not going to get the results. And vice versa. The nutrition part is 60 to 70 percent of it."

The basic premise of the diet, which Isaacs prescribes to all of his clients, is eating balanced meals consisting of whole foods, and the less processed, the better. "You want to eat as close to the farm, as close to nature, as possible," Isaacs says. These types of foods are highly nutritious and will fill you up on fewer calories.

About 60 percent of your calories should come from complex carbohydrates (vegetables, whole grains, fruits), 20 percent from fat (olive or canola oil, nuts, or avocado), and 20 percent from lean protein (chicken, turkey, fish). Fish may actually be one of the better sources of protein. A small preliminary study found that consuming three to six ounces of fish a day may help you burn more fat and lose more weight even if you're eating the same number of calories as you did previously.

Normally, the recommendation for a healthy diet is 10 to 15 percent of calories from protein, but this diet is a bit higher. There is some evidence suggesting that people who exercise hard may need more protein than average Joes and Janes.

The exercise portion is based on the program that got Melanie Griffith back in shape after the birth of her daughter Stella last year, and it's what can get you to drop a size this month. Before you jump to the diet and exercise charts, you need to understand the key concepts of success.

Progress is key. Over the course of four weeks, your workouts will increase in length and your menus will offer more variety. The first week, you'll have few food choices, making what you're going to eat one less thing to worry about. But as the weeks go by and you regain control of your eating habits, you'll have more options to choose from.

Keep challenging your muscles. This is your exercise objective. When muscles get used to one activity, they get really good at it. In other words, it becomes easy, so you burn fewer calories. Aerobic goal: To keep your muscles at maximum burning capacity, you need to mix up the types of aerobic activity that you do during a week. Every week, increase the length of your workouts to burn even more calories, and even at the longest, the workout is done in less than an hour a day. Strength training goal: Increase the amount of weight you're lifting each week. Weights should be heavy enough that after 15 repetitions, you couldn't do another one even for $100. If you can, increase the weight.

Dine on mini-meals. When Melanie Griffith is getting ready for a photo shoot or a movie, she eats five small meals throughout the day. Try this. The mini-meals will help keep your blood sugar levels on an even keel, so you'll avoid late-morning or late-afternoon slumps. It will also feel like you're eating more, so you won't be hungry. One small study showed that boxers eating six small meals a day burned more fat than boxers eating the same number of calories a day in only two meals. Since the total number of calories you eat is still most important in weight control, just remember to keep portions under control so you don't eat too many calories.

Keep your portion sizes in check. When it comes to plain fruits and vegetables, you can eat to your heart's content. But you need to keep an eye on portion sizes when you're eating other types of foods. If you're having pasta, rice, beans, or cereals as a main dish, don't eat more than one cup—and only serve a half-cup if you're having these foods as side dishes. Having some bread? Limit yourself to one slice. And if you want a bagel, cut it in half and save the other half for tomorrow. Servings of meat or fish should be no larger than three ounces, which is about the size of a deck of cards. And when you dip into any kind of spread—apple butter, jelly, peanut butter, or cottage cheese—don't take more than a tablespoon.

Focus on shorter, faster workouts. You're going to push yourself a little harder, but don't worry. You'll be amazed at how much your body can do. And you'll feel more invigorated for doing it.

The trick is to get out of your comfort zone and work at an intensity at which you find it difficult to carry on a conversation, but you are still able to respond in short phrases. "If you can have a conversation comfortably while you're doing your cardio workout, you're not burning the correct number of calories," Isaacs says. Sure, you could burn the same number of calories by exercising longer, but who has the time? Plus, the higher intensity will keep your body's calorie-burning engine revving high for longer after you stop exercising.

Sundays are freebies. You'll notice that there are no meal plans for Sundays. That's your day to kick back and eat what you want (within reason). Go out for brunch or dinner and order pancakes, a burger, frozen yogurt, or a slice of pie for a treat. These foods aren't forbidden; you just don't want to eat them regularly. Allowing yourself some planned indulgences may help keep your cravings under control throughout the rest of the week.

Although this is designed as a four-week program, don't just go back to your old habits at the end of the month. That's a surefire way to regain all the lost pounds and inches. Instead, continue with the basic program and see even better results. Now it's time to take control of your body. A month from now, you'll be impressed.

Working Out with Melanie Griffith

Actress Melanie Griffith is living proof that Greg Isaacs' program is effective. "Whatever Greg says, do it because it really, really works!" she says.

Her usual routine is a half-hour run, a half-hour on the stairclimber, and abdominal exercises. Her favorite workout, though, is a long hike. "It's more enjoyable being outside where it's really beautiful or having a goal to climb to the top of a hill." (For strength-training exercises, you'll want to have the advice of a trainer or physical therapist to demonstrate the correct positions and make sure you're doing them correctly.)

She also makes time for healthy eating. Griffith sticks to Isaacs' rule of eating whole, natural foods. Fruits and veggies are her staples, along with some fish and chicken and an occasional indulgence in spareribs.

WEEK 1

Monday
Exercise: walk or run (18 to 20 minutes)
Breakfast: oatmeal made with fat-free milk; grapefruit or melon
Snack: apples, melon, kiwifruit, pineapple, or mango with nonfat yogurt
Lunch: tuna sandwich with fat-free mayonnaise on whole-grain bread; fat-free lentil soup; salad with fat-free dressing
Snack: baked tortilla chips with salsa
Dinner: baked potato topped with fat-free cheese and mushrooms sautéed in broth and low-sodium soy sauce; steamed veggies

Tuesday
Exercise: ride a stationary bike (18 to 20 minutes)
Breakfast: fruit bowl (melons, bananas, and kiwifruit topped with fat-free yogurt or fat-free cottage cheese); fat-free, low-sugar muffin
Snack: high-fiber cereal with fat-free milk
Lunch: steamed veggies over brown rice with salsa or low-sodium soy sauce; salad with low-fat dressing
Dinner: grilled or baked fish or chicken; steamed veggies

Wednesday
Exercise: strength training—crunches, squats, pelvic tilts, chest presses, bent-over rows, shoulder presses, bicep curls, tricep kickbacks
Same menu as Monday

Thursday

> *Exercise:* aerobics class or video (18 to 20 minutes)
>
> *Same menu as Tuesday*

Friday

> *Exercise:* walk or run (18 to 20 minutes)
>
> *Same menu as Monday*

Saturday

> *Exercise:* strength training (same as Wednesday)
>
> *Same menu as Tuesday*

Sunday

> *Exercise:* yoga (45 minutes)
>
> *Take the day off from menus*

WEEK 2

Monday

> *Exercise:* walk or run (20 to 30 minutes)
>
> *Breakfast:* egg-white omelet with tomatoes, spinach, mushrooms, and salsa; toast or bagel with jelly
>
> *Snack:* fat-free yogurt
>
> *Lunch:* pizza (light on the cheese) topped with veggies; salad with fat-free dressing
>
> *Snack:* fat-free hearty soup (lentil, vegetable, bean, or pea)
>
> *Dinner:* chicken stir-fry with veggies over rice

Tuesday

> *Exercise:* ride a stationary bike (20 to 30 minutes)
>
> *Breakfast:* whole-wheat pancakes with fruit syrup; nonfat yogurt
>
> *Snack:* raw veggies with salsa
>
> *Lunch:* grilled chicken breast or turkey burger on whole-wheat roll with mustard, lettuce, and tomato; salad with fat-free dressing
>
> *Snack:* air-popped popcorn with rice vinegar or spices
>
> *Dinner:* vegetarian chili with whole-grain bread

Wednesday

> *Exercise:* strength training—repeat exercises from week 1 and add lower-ab leg lifts (single leg, not double from back lying position), chest flies, pullovers, lateral raises, hammer curls, bench dips
>
> *Choose meals from weeks 1 or 2*

Thursday

> *Exercise:* aerobics class or video (20 to 30 minutes)
>
> *Choose meals from weeks 1 or 2*

(continued)

Working Out with Melanie Griffith
—Continued

Friday
  Exercise: walk or run (20 to 30 minutes)
  Choose meals from weeks 1 or 2
Saturday
  Exercise: strength training (same as Wednesday)
  Choose meals from weeks 1 or 2
Sunday
  Exercise: yoga (45 minutes)
  Take the day off from menus

WEEK 3

Monday
  Exercise: walk or run (30 to 40 minutes)
  Breakfast: fresh fruit smoothie; bagel with fat-free cottage cheese
  Snack: rice cakes with reduced-fat peanut butter
  Lunch: pasta with red sauce and veggies; salad with fat-free
    dressing; whole-grain bread
  Snack: fat-free pretzels
  Dinner: green peppers stuffed with lean turkey and rice; fruit
Tuesday
  Exercise: ride a stationary bike (20 to 30 minutes)
  Breakfast: fat-free granola with nonfat yogurt and fruit
  Snack: bagel with fat-free cream cheese and tomato
  Lunch: grilled chicken salad with chickpeas and fat-free dressing
  Snack: fruit
  Dinner: fat-free soup (bean, lentil, pea, or vegetable); salad with
    fat-free dressing; whole-grain roll
Wednesday
  Exercise: strength training—repeat exercises from week 2 and add
    walking, lunges, pushups, pullovers, seated back laterals,
    frontal raises
  Choose meals from weeks 1, 2, or 3
Thursday
  Exercise: aerobics class or video (30 to 40 minutes)
  Choose meals from weeks 1, 2, or 3

Friday
> *Exercise:* walk or run (30 to 40 minutes)
> *Choose meals from weeks 1, 2, or 3*

Saturday
> *Exercise:* strength training (same as Wednesday)
> *Choose meals from weeks 1, 2, or 3*

Sunday
> *Exercise:* yoga (45 minutes)
> *Take the day off from menus*

WEEK 4

Monday
> *Exercise:* walk or run (45 minutes)
> *Breakfast:* high-fiber cereal with fat-free milk
> *Snack:* fruit
> *Lunch:* turkey sandwich on whole-wheat bread with mustard, lettuce, and tomato; fat-free soup
> *Snack:* choose from previous options
> *Dinner:* stir-fried vegetables over rice; salad with fat-free dressing

Tuesday
> *Exercise:* ride a stationary bike (45 minutes)
> *Choose meals from weeks 1, 2, or 3*

Wednesday
> *Exercise:* strength training—repeat exercises from week 3 and do an extra set of each
> *Choose meals from weeks 1, 2, or 3*

Thursday
> *Exercise:* aerobics class or video (45 minutes)
> *Choose meals from weeks 1, 2, or 3*

Friday
> *Exercise:* walk or run (45 minutes)
> *Choose meals from weeks 1, 2, or 3*

Saturday
> *Exercise:* strength training (same as Wednesday)
> *Choose meals from weeks 1, 2, or 3*

Sunday
> *Exercise:* yoga (45 minutes)
> *Take the day off from menus*

71 Weight-Loss Tips That Really Work

Want to get the real scoop on losing weight? How to take it off and keep it off for good?

The editors of *Prevention* magazine wanted to know what really worked for folks who had not only lost big pounds (more than 30), but who had kept it off for more than a year. The 71 answers here came from people who have shared their experiences with others through the National Weight Control Registry. Here's the advice of more than two dozen members—along with other vets of weight loss.

Not surprisingly, they changed their eating habits and increased their activity levels. But haven't we all tried that? Why did it work for them and not others? Here is their advice.

Get Moving

The tough part with exercise, of course, is getting out there and doing it. Here's how they get going.

1. Prioritize. The beds might not get made, but Amy Reed, 36, still makes time for exercise. That's how she has kept off more than 80 pounds for 13 years. "I have to schedule it in and let go of other things, like a perfectly clean house," she says.

2. Find a passion. "I have a dance background and when I found jazzercise, I said, 'Thank God.' If somebody had told me I had to go out and run five days a week, I'd still weigh 185 pounds," says Anne Geren, 41, who lost 55 pounds and has kept it off for 13 years.

3. Keep an exercise log. It makes you more accountable. Norma from Dallas, who hangs hers on the refrigerator, checks off six workouts a week dutifully. "If I miss one day, I make that my day off for the week."

4. Set a goal. Sign up for some fun runs and try to improve your times. "I went from a 5-K to a 4-miler, then a 5-miler, then a 10-K. As I was building miles and speed, I was getting fitter and losing more weight," says Therese Revitt, 42, who lost 80 pounds and recently ran a marathon.

5. Get pumped. "It wasn't until I put on more muscle through resistance training that I was able to keep the weight off almost effortlessly," says Verona Mucci-Hurlburt, 37, who went from a size 18 to an 8. The reason? Muscle burns more calories around the clock.

Eat Smart

6. Make changes for the long haul. "I learned how to eat and live with it for the rest of my life," says Barbara Miltenberger, 42, who lost more than 40 pounds and hasn't seen any come back in three years.

7. Stop dieting. "The best thing I did was quit dieting," says Reed. "I'd always find ways to cheat. So instead, I stopped forbidding myself certain foods and just started eating less of them."

8. Get a grip on reality. "When I started keeping a food diary, I discovered that I was eating somewhere between 3,000 and 4,000 calories a day," says Rebecca, 46, who found the number shocking.

9. Eat mini-meals. Having smaller, more frequent meals can prevent you from getting ravenously hungry and overeating. On average, weight-loss winners eat five times a day.

10. Follow the 90 percent to 10 percent rule. "If you watch what you eat 90 percent of the time, the other 10 percent is not a problem," says Mucci-Hurlburt, who learned this tip from a fitness professional.

11. Dine at the dinner table only. If you eat in front of the TV, then every time you nestle in with the remote control, it's a cue to eat. Instead, designate an eating spot for all meals and snacks. "Even when I want potato chips, I set the table just as if I was going to sit down for a full-course meal," says Kathy Wilson, 47, who took off more than 100 pounds. "I put a handful of chips on the plate, put the bag away, and then sit down to eat. I never just stand at the counter and eat now."

12. Think before you bite. Creating rituals like Wilson did or the old standby of waiting 10 minutes before giving in to a craving can stop you from eating when you really aren't hungry. "Nine chances out of 10, the chips go back in the cupboard, and I just walk away," says Wilson.

13. Drink up. "Drinking lots of water keeps me from snacking when I'm not hungry, and it gives me more energy," says Revitt. "It also stopped what I thought were hunger headaches, which were probably due to dehydration."

Set Yourself Up for Success

14. Do it for yourself. "My doctor told me for years that I had to take the weight off. But you have to want it yourself," says Wilson.

"As long as somebody else is pushing you, no matter what you do or what you try, it'll never work," adds Victoria Bennett, 39, who shed 60 pounds and has kept them off for five years.

15. Take it slow. We all want to lose it yesterday, but slow is the way to go if you don't want to see those pounds again. "It took me a year to lose 100 pounds this time," says Rebecca, who has kept it off for eight years. "I had lost 100 pounds twice before, in less than six months each time, but I didn't maintain it."

16. Customize your approach. What worked for your best friend may not work for you. And what works for you today may not work six months from now. You need to decide what you need. Mucci-Hurlburt joined a structured program for accountability. "I needed to know that I was going to get weighed each week," she says. But for others, that's exactly what they don't need.

17. Learn from the past. Everyone we talked to had tried to lose weight before. Part of their success this time was that they learned from past failures. "Before, the more I focused on weighing, measuring, and preparing food, the more I ate," says Wilson, who finally succeeded with a program that offered prepackaged foods.

18. Set small goals. "My first goal was to lose only 10 pounds," says Rebecca. "I had very high blood pressure, and my doctor said that if I would just lose 10 pounds, he believed that I could get off the pills. Every other doctor before said I had to lose 100 pounds, and I thought 'I can't do that.' But 10 pounds, I thought, 'Maybe I can do that.' Doing it one bite at a time made it more achievable for me."

19. Make changes you can live with. "Before I'd go to bed I'd ask myself, 'Is what I did today something I could do for the rest of my life?' If I felt deprived, I'd do it differently tomorrow. If I thought, 'Yeah, I could do this tomorrow,' then I was on the right track," says Revitt.

Control Portions

20. Go back to school. Joining a weight-loss class or working with a dietitian can help you learn proper portions, even without weighing and measuring. "If you get a half-cup of cottage cheese, it should look like a tennis ball; a quarter-cup should look like a Ping-Pong ball," says Wilson. "Now, I know what appropriate portions look like."

21. Don't toss those measuring cups, though. "I usually mis-

Five Meals in Minutes . . . Really

In a rush? These quick meals are great for eating healthy in a hurry.

Fast wraps. Wrap beans, grated low-fat cheese, rice, and salsa in a tortilla for a low-fat burrito. Add a side of crunchy baby carrots for a complete meal.

Quick potatoes. Toss a sweet potato in the microwave for six to nine minutes. Stuff it with precut vegetables and grated low-fat cheese and add a dessert of fresh-cut fruit.

Instant lunch. Not much fills you up better or faster than instant bean or lentil soup, says Dayle Hayes, R.D., a nutrition consultant in Billings, Montana, and author of *Moving Away from Diets*. Soup and breadsticks make it a quick lunch.

Pronto pasta. Couscous cooks in five minutes. Try this nutty pasta with fresh-cut fruit in the morning, stuffed in a pita with beans and grated low-fat cheese for lunch, or with canned chicken and heated vegetables for dinner.

Quickest chicken. Sauté precut chicken and vegetables in canola oil and low-sodium soy sauce. Pour over instant rice for a low-fat stir-fry.

judge portions of salad dressing, mayonnaise, and ice cream," says Revitt. "They're really high in fat and calories and cause the most damage if overdone. So I still measure them."

22. Cook for your family, not an army. Even for low-fat foods like grilled chicken, Bennett stopped overfeeding her family of four. "I stopped making six or seven breasts, thinking that everybody had to have two or three," she says. "Now, I make just one for each person."

Take Some Cooking Lessons

23. Plan ahead. An empty fridge after a stressful day begs for pizza. The now-slender crew doesn't leave meals to chance. Many of them plan their menus a week or more in advance. Others even cook ahead, freezing meals for the week in individual containers.

24. A little dab will do it. If you just can't pass on some high-fat favorites, stick to the most flavorful ones. "A single slice of bacon is enough to flavor eggs or a potato," says Helen Fitzgerald, 61, who lost about 51 pounds. Her husband has lost more than 150 pounds.

25. Fake fry. Try "frying" with calorie-free cooking sprays instead of oil. Spray sliced potatoes and roast them in the oven for french fries that taste fried without the fat, suggests Miltenberger.

26. Stock frozen veggies. With pasta or stir-fry sauces, they are diet saviors. "I've been known to eat a whole bag of vegetables, and with only a quarter-cup of sauce, it's only about three grams of fat," says Mucci-Hurlburt. "It has saved my butt many times when I was really hungry and had to eat now."

27. Flavor up. Rice, beans, and other cooked grains are the staples of many successful dieters. For variety, Fitzgerald cooks them in different liquids, such as tomato juice, apple juice, or beef or chicken stock. "Rice done in pineapple juice is especially good for rice puddings and Chinese-style dishes," she says.

Don't Go It Alone

28. Find the right support person. A nag won't do. Neither will a partner in crime. Look for someone who can empathize and support you in a positive way. When Reed finally succeeded in losing weight, her fiancé was a big help. "We didn't focus all our socializing around food. We went bike riding a lot and played tennis instead of going for pizza."

29. Join a support group. "Hearing someone say she lost 50 pounds would be real motivating," says Revitt. "I'd think, 'She's just a normal person like me. If she can lose 50, then I can do it, too.'"

30. Create your own group. "I started my first women's group when I first started exercising. It was just a bunch of women who got together once a week, and we would compare notes," says Debra Mazda, 44, who is 135 pounds slimmer than she was 13 years ago.

Don't Boycott Dining Out

31. Be picky. "I'm not afraid to ask for dishes to be prepared differently," says Bennett. "My philosophy is that every restaurant has a grill and an oven. They don't have to fry everything."

32. It's not the Last Supper. This is not your last chance in life to have a particular food. "Those french fries will be there in a half-hour if I really have to have them," says Mucci-Hurlburt. Or they'll be there next week.

Smart Tips for Snacking

There's a lot to be said for eating when you're hungry—but that doesn't mean you always want to give in to a snack attack. Here are some guideposts along the treacherous road of snacking.

- Buy a healthy afternoon snack along with your lunch. That way you won't be tempted by fatty stuff when you make another trip to the cafeteria or vending machines.
- Vow that each time you eat—especially if it's an unplanned snack—to first enjoy a piece of fruit or a vegetable.
- When a craving hits, try brushing your teeth or rinsing with mouthwash. This can help if you just can't keep your hand out of the bag of chips, even though you tucked it way back in the cupboard.
- Make a snack food that you're craving part of a regular meal. You'll be less likely to binge on it later.

33. Don't wait to doggie bag. "As soon as the waitress puts the food down in front of me, I cut the whole portion in half, put half on my butter plate, and ask her to wrap it," says Revitt. If you wait until the end of your meal, often you pick at it until the waitress returns.

34. Tackle buffets. "I get only one tablespoon of everything," says Rebecca. "Usually, I don't even fill my plate, but I at least taste everything so I don't feel deprived."

Deliver Yourself from Temptation

35. Stay busy. Do something that's not conducive to eating. The go-getters in the weight-loss club aren't sitting around thinking of hot-fudge sundaes. They're singing in choirs, taking classes, running marathons, leading weight-loss groups, and more.

36. Keep 'em out of sight. Overwhelmingly, weight-loss vets control foods like chocolate, ice cream, and potato chips by not having them around. "It's easier to fill the house with treats for my kids if I choose ones that I don't like, such as Oreo cookies," says 30-year-old Tammy Hansen, who trimmed off 60 pounds.

37. Moderation is key. Weight-loss vets aren't depriving themselves, either. "If I want a piece of cake, I'll have one," says Mazda. "Then I just won't have another one for a week or so. Knowing that I can eat something and no one is going to say 'you can't' works for me."

38. Indulge and enjoy. Go for the best brand of ice cream or the best cut of steak. "If I'm going to blow 500 or 600 calories, I want to make sure that I'm enjoying it to the max," says Mucci-Hurlburt. "Often, desserts look much better than they taste. If it tastes like cardboard, forget it. It's not worth it."

39. Limit portions. "When I have to snack, I put my hand in the bag or box and whatever I can grab, that's what I eat—only a handful," says Fitzgerald.

40. Buy individually packaged snacks. Cookies, chips, even ice cream come in single-serving sizes. "If I want some cookies or chips, I grab one little bag instead of a whole box," says Reed.

41. Keep reminders around. A note on the refrigerator reading "Stop" kept Reed from raiding it. Underneath, she listed other things to do, like "Take a drink of water," and questions such as "Are you really hungry?"

42. Find alternatives. Chocolate is still a favorite even for successful dieters. But they've found ways to enjoy it and still keep their waistlines. Bennett makes fat-free chocolate pudding with skim milk.

For Sarah, who lost 40 pounds and has kept it off for two years, a cup of fat-free, sugar-free hot cocoa (about 20 calories), topped with a little fat-free whipped cream, does the trick.

43. Don't give in to peer pressure. If the cookies, chips, or ice cream treats that you buy for the rest of the family are sabotaging your efforts, stop buying it. "My daughters carried on for about a month, but after that, they got used to the change," says Bennett.

Escape Emotional Eating

44. Know your triggers. You have to know which moods send you to the cookie jar before you can do anything about it. Once you know your triggers, have a list of alternate things to do when the mood strikes. "When I get tired or discouraged, I get an 'I don't care attitude,'" says Rebecca. For those times, taking a walk or reading affirmations can help.

45. Quiz yourself. Determine if you're really hungry or if you're eating for other reasons. "I'll ask myself 'Do I really want this, or is it something else, like boredom or depression?' About 80 percent of the time, it's not hunger," says Geren.

46. Call a friend. Talking about what's eating you can keep you from eating. "I had to be willing to call my support people at nine o'clock on a Friday night," says Barbara, 46, who has kept off 46 pounds for more than 15 years.

47. Stop worrying. Remind yourself that you only have control over yourself, not over your spouse, boss, parents, or friends. If you can't do anything about it, just let it go, several people suggest.

48. Take an emotional inventory. Ask yourself, "What do I feel guilty about? Resent? Fear? Regret? What am I angry about?" Then deal with it, says Barbara. Confront the person involved, talk to others, or write a letter even if you don't send it.

49. Get spiritual. If religion isn't for you, try yoga, meditation, or relaxation exercises. These are especially helpful if you tend to eat when you're stressed, says Barbara.

50. Challenge the power of food. Ice cream is a poor companion if you're lonely. "If I eat the whole bag of chocolate chip cookies, am I going to be any happier? Probably not," says Wilson.

Blast Off a Plateau

51. Up the ante. "I started out walking, and eventually tried running, which was the key to my success," says Revitt. "I couldn't even make it around one lap (1/26 of a mile) in the beginning, but it was just enough to make the weight loss continue."

52. Go back to basics. "I'd go back to more strict measuring because you can sneak away from reasonable portions and start fooling yourself," says Mucci-Hurlburt.

53. Stop starving yourself. "As soon as I saw the weight coming off, I thought, 'If it's working at this rate, I'll try eating less so I'll lose more,'" admits Miltenberger. "Then I'd stall or even put weight on because I was undereating and my metabolism slowed. I'd start losing again when I'd eat a little bit more."

54. Look how far you've come. "By keeping a graph of my weight, I could see that the line would go up and down and up and down, but overall it was going down, so there was no reason to throw away my progress," says Rebecca.

Stay Motivated

55. Don't give up. "There have been plenty of times when I have wanted to give up, but I didn't," says Mazda. "I realized a long time ago that entrepreneurs fall and rise up every time they lose a venture, but they just keep getting up." The same is true for weight loss.

56. "You can do it." Repeat this to yourself. Many people post affirmations around their homes or offices as constant reminders. One dieter even programmed her computer screen to keep her on the right track.

57. Get inspired. "I read a lot about other people who have come back from obstacles and really made it," says Mazda. Their determination can make you feel like you can succeed, too.

58. Envision your svelte self. "If you can actually visualize yourself as the person you want to be, you'll become her," says Wilson. "When I felt like I couldn't do this one more minute, I slipped in a motivational tape. Step by step, it would walk me through a visualization exercise so I could see myself as I wanted to be."

59. Find new measures of success. When she lost some weight, trying on her old, too-big clothes further motivated Miltenberger. "I also bought myself a size below what I was wearing," she says. "I'd see if I could get the pants on, then if I could zip them and, finally, when I could wear them comfortably."

Feel Good about Yourself

60. Learn to like your trouble spots. Peggy Malecha, who has lost about 75 pounds, dresses in a black leotard and, standing in front of a mirror, she points out everything about herself that she doesn't like. Then she counters that. For instance, "I hate my legs, but they work," she says. "I can walk and dance. I have no control over the way they look, so it's silly to obsess over them. Don't dwell on it."

61. Pamper yourself. Take baths and get massages, facials, manicures, and pedicures. "They make me look good and feel good," says Mazda.

62. Stop negative talk. "If you make positive speech a long-term goal and stop using 'I was bad (or good) today,' you'll begin to feel better about yourself," says Mazda.

63. Don't compare yourself with others. "Instead, think, 'I'm better or just as good as anyone else is.' Once you start thinking that about yourself, believe me, you get real cocky," says Mazda.

64. Look in the mirror and say, "I look good." You may not believe it now, but you will. "When I first started this, I avoided mirrors," says Bennett. "I never wanted to go into a dressing room, so I'd get various sizes, take them home, and then try them on. If they didn't fit, then I took them back. But now, I'll look in every mirror."

Be Realistic

65. Stay flexible. Many people who have kept the weight off never reached their initial goal weights. Instead, they've gotten to a realistic weight that they can maintain. "In 13 years, I've never gotten down to my initial goal weight, but I'm very happy and feel very good even though I didn't reach it," says Reed.

66. Quit the numbers game. Mucci-Hurlburt is 5 feet 5½ inches tall and weighs 152 pounds. By society's standards, she's heavy. However, she can slip into a size eight thanks to the fact that most of her weight is muscle. "It doesn't matter what the scale says; it matters how I look," she says.

67. Reject others' standards. "Thin is whatever you think thin is. Next to Roseanne, I'm thin. Next to Twiggy, I'm fat," says Mazda.

Get Back on Track

68. Stop being a perfectionist. "Look at it like walking a tightrope," suggests Revitt. "The goal is not just to stay on without falling off. The goal is to get to the other side, and if you know that you can fall off as many times as you want as long as you get back on again, you're going to be successful."

69. Start fresh, ASAP. If you slip, don't wait until Monday or even tomorrow to get back in line. Revitt uses water as a cleansing ritual to end a binge. When she realizes what's happening, she drinks water to signal that the eating is over, and she's back on track immediately. "It has made my lapses shorter and shorter," she says.

70. Practice early detection. "I weigh myself about once a month," says Reed. "If I start inching up, I increase my exercise a little bit."

71. Enlist professional help. Many people use dietitians, personal trainers, and even psychologists to help them deal with problems that hinder their weight-loss efforts. If you feel like you can't do it on your own, seek help.

17 Ways to Restart Stalled Weight Loss

So you're still doing the same things that peeled off the first 5, 10, or 50 pounds. You've kept up the daily walk, and you're a role model for low-fat eating. So why does it seem that your scale is stuck?

You're on a plateau. Join the club. It happens to people losing weight all the time. "Plateaus can happen when you're doing the same thing as you always were, diet- and exercise-wise," says Terri Brownlee, R.D., a dietitian at the Duke University Diet and Fitness Center in Durham, North Carolina.

What's changed is you.

The smaller you are, the fewer calories you require. So the diet and exercise program that helped you get from 190 pounds down to 160 may not be burning enough calories to get you to your goal of 145.

This doesn't mean that you have to swear off satisfying meals or walk to the other side of the state and back to get rid of more pounds. You just need to stop for a minute and grab a pencil.

1. Keep a positive attitude. "Instead of getting down on yourself, try to understand what's not working and rethink your strategy," says Cathy Nonas, R.D., administrative director of the Theodore B. VanItallie Center for Nutrition and Weight Management at St. Luke's–Roosevelt Hospital in New York City.

That's what Cathy Upchurch did when she hit a two-month plateau after losing 70 pounds. "I kept on giving myself pep talks and refused to give up," says this 45-year-old Colorado work-at-home woman. "I kept telling myself that I was an athletic person underneath it all and that there were all these fun things I wanted to do." She eventually lost another 70 pounds and has kept it all off for eight years. Like her, thousands of people have come up against plateaus and been victorious. You can too.

2. Meet the challenges head-on. As important as a positive attitude is, you need specific and careful evaluation, as well. "Once you see what the problems are, you can get back on track," says Pamela Walker, Ph.D., a clinical psychologist at the Cooper Aerobics Center in Dallas. "It shifts the focus from 'something is wrong with me' to problem solving."

3. Contend with complacency. The first thing you want to take a look at is what you're eating and doing. Have your portions expanded

Is It Really a Plateau or Your Ideal Weight?

If you're still 70 pounds more than what most weight tables recommend for your height, chances are, you're just on a plateau. If you're merely 10 pounds more, then it might be time to accept your weight. In between? That's a gray area.

Ideal weight varies among individuals. If you're in that gray area, here are things to consider when deciding if you should lose more weight.

- Are you weight training? Muscle weighs more than fat but looks a heck of a lot better.
- Where's the weight? If those stubborn pounds are around your middle, they could be increasing your risk of heart disease, diabetes, and even some types of cancer. You're at greater risk if you're or a man or a premenopausal woman under the age of forty and your waist is greater than 39 inches. If you're over 40, you have a higher risk of these health problems—whether you're a man or a premenopausal woman—if your waist is over 35 inches. And if you're a woman who's over 40 and also past menopause, you're at greater risk if your waist is larger than 33 inches.
- Do you have any signs of high cholesterol, high blood pressure, or high blood sugar? These may be the first clues that your weight is affecting your health.
- Is it realistic to eat any less or exercise any more?

"You can't diet forever," says David Levitsky, Ph.D., professor of nutrition and psychology at Cornell University in Ithaca, New York. "It's better to choose a lifestyle that encourages healthy weight and in which exercise and healthy eating are a regular part of the program than to obsess over a few pounds."

Balancing Act

The slimmer you get, the less effective your current weight-loss plan will be. Here's why.

If you are a woman who weighed 190 pounds and you were sedentary when you started, you burned 2,280 calories a day to maintain that weight. (For men, the calorie burn is slightly more.) If you ate 2,280 calories and burned 344 calories in a one-hour walk, you burned 344 calories more than your body needed to maintain that weight, so you lost weight.

Say you reach 160 pounds. Now, you need only 1,920 calories to stay at your current weight. But you're still eating 2,280 calories and going for a one-hour walk. Since you're lighter, your walk burns 292 calories. Now you're eating 68 calories more than you're burning. Keep it up, and the scale will start moving in the wrong direction.

Here's how it adds up.

If you weigh 190 and you eat:	2,280 calories
You burn*:	-2,280 calories
You exercise:	-344 calories
Result:	-344 calories a day and weight loss

If you weigh 160 and you eat:	2,280 calories
You burn*:	-1,920 calories
You exercise:	-292 calories
Result:	+68 calories a day

This means a plateau, even though your eating and exercising habits haven't changed. Over time, you'll regain some weight unless you shift the balance.

*To maintain your current weight if you're sedentary

as your waistline has shrunk? "Many people who experience success start getting overconfident and complacent," Dr. Walker says. "Portions start creeping up, and sweets are slowly added again."

4. Put exercise in the driver's seat. Has your exercise routine taken a backseat to less strenuous activity? Exercise is always one of the first things to go. Walks get shorter or get skipped.

Careful examination of eating and exercise logs can pinpoint areas where your guard may be down. Skipping your evening workout in favor of drinks with friends, or indulging your sweet tooth more frequently? No time to pack a healthy lunch, so you're resorting to the vending machines?

"It makes you accountable to yourself, and frequently, you're shocked to see that you did start eating more and exercising less," Dr. Walker says.

5. Get calories under control. No matter how you got on the plateau, the answer to blasting off it is to shake things up. You need to start burning more calories than you're taking in.

6. Measure your portions. Arm yourself with measuring devices like scales or cups so you don't have to rely on your eyes (or your stomach), says Nonas. Once you're familiar with what your portion sizes should be, you need only measure from time to time to make sure that you're still on track. Keep portions reasonable. (But don't put limits on plain veggies, raw or cooked. And try for three to five servings of fruit a day.)

7. Shortcut portion control. Stock up on prepackaged low-fat meals. Food labels make it easy to know exactly what you're getting, and you save yourself the job of measuring portions.

8. Try a meal substitute. Liquid meals can be helpful, especially when you're on the run. This shouldn't become a long-term strategy, but it can help break a plateau.

9. Fill up on whole foods. Bananas, carrots, and air-popped popcorn pack more fiber and fewer calories than reduced-fat cakes or cookies, so you feel full on less food.

10. Postpone dinner. Eating half an hour or even an hour later than usual may be just what you need to take the edge off late-night munchies.

11. Drink up. "Put a liter of water on your desk, and make sure you drink it by the end of the day," says Nonas. Filling up on water during the day can help make portion control easier at meals.

12. Limit meal times. So you stuck to your portion, but then you ate your kids' leftovers, and before you knew it, you were noshing ad infinitum. "It's important to do things that signal the end of the meal, like brushing your teeth," says Nonas.

13. Burn more calories; add a minute. "Gradually extend the length of your workouts," says J. P. Slovak, fitness director at the Cooper Fitness Center in Dallas. A few extra minutes here and there can go a long way toward producing real results.

14. Lift some weights. To combat the decrease in metabolism that often comes with weight loss, increase your muscle mass. Muscles burn more calories than fat, even when you're sleeping. And they take up less space, so you look slimmer.

15. Try something new. You're not the only one who gets bored on the stationary bike—your muscles do, too. If you always work the same muscles in the same way, they become very efficient and then won't burn as many calories as when you first started doing the activity, explains Tedd Mitchell, M.D., medical director at the Cooper Wellness Program in Dallas. If you want to shake up your metabolism, work your muscles in new ways by cross-training. If you're walking, try swimming. If you're running, try boxing. No one activity should ever get to be too easy.

16. Add some intervals. Invigorate your routine with short blasts of very intense exercise. "Try not to mosey along at the same pace," says Dr. Mitchell. "Sprint for an interval if you're running. Pedal really fast on the bike if you're cycling." Intervals not only make working out more exciting and challenging, they also help burn extra calories.

17. Go the long way. "You don't need to have gym clothes on to get exercise," says Kyle McInnis, Ph.D., professor in the department of human performance and fitness at the University of Massachusetts in Boston. Use the second-floor bathroom or the copier down the hall. "Accumulating physical activity throughout the day, such as walking more and taking the stairs, adds up," he says.

Get the Body You Want, Even If You Can't Lose Weight

After losing 20 pounds, 43-year-old Judy McCoy was still unhappy with her body. In fact, it wasn't until she stopped losing weight that she finally got the body she wanted.

In only six months, McCoy firmed up and slimmed down. She lost more than three inches off her upper arms and thighs, more than four inches from her hips, nearly five inches off her waist, and dropped one size. "I didn't lose any weight," she says. "I just redistributed it. My husband said he felt like he was living with Cindy Crawford."

McCoy is not the only one to have transformed her body even

when the scale was barely moving. At age 42, Susan Flagg Godbey had to give away her favorite clothes because they were too tight. A year later, she was buying clothes two sizes smaller, but she had only lost six pounds. "I felt like I could wear anything, even cropped workout tops that exposed my waist," she says, adding that after she had a baby five years earlier, she thought she'd never have a flat stomach again.

What's their secret? It's simple and much easier than you think. It's weight training. Lifting weights is the best and quickest way to shape up your body. "If you work out consistently for 30 minutes three days a week, you'll feel stronger in two weeks and look more toned in six to eight weeks," says Chester Zelasko, Ph.D., chairman of the health and wellness department at Buffalo State College in New York.

The first spots to show improvement are those with the least body fat, usually your upper back and arms, says Karen Andes, a San Francisco personal trainer and author of *A Woman's Book of Strength*. Andes notes that a woman's chest will get stronger, which helps hold her breasts a little higher. The abs and legs are the slowest to show changes.

"I started strength training when I hit 37 and found that I couldn't lose weight as easily as I used to," says businesswoman Pati deVries Ames, who has been lifting weights for about six months. "My energy level just shot up, and within two months my body was really toned, especially my arms."

Still have half a dozen excuses for not starting? Here are just some of the excuses that crop up most often among women who avoid strength training. (Men use some of these excuses, of course—and other ones, too.) Want to listen in on the inner debate? Read on.

Excuse: "I have to lose weight first."

Reality: "I call that the 'cleaning up for the maid syndrome,'" says Andes. "Women think that they have to get thin before they can go to the gym. But strength training is a good way to start exercising. You see a more overall conditioning than you would with, say, walking, which mostly exercises the legs. And resistance workouts can help you get the strength you may need to sustain aerobic workouts."

One added bonus is that the more muscle you have, the higher your metabolism—the rate at which your body burns calories. This is especially important since everyone begins to experience a decline in metabolism of about 0.5 percent every year after age 25. That's one reason why it gets harder to stay thin as you get older. But lifting weights and building muscle can reverse that. According to Wayne Westcott, Ph.D., *Prevention*'s strength-training advisor, strength consultant to the YMCA of the USA, and author of *Strength Training Past 50*, you can increase your resting metabolic rate by 7 percent after just three months of regular weight training, which will help you lose weight.

Weight training has payoffs beyond aesthetics, too. It helps prevent osteoporosis (the bone-thinning disease), reverses the loss in strength that happens after age 25, lowers the risk of adult-onset diabetes, decreases resting blood pressure, improves lower-back problems, and reduces the pain of arthritis, Dr. Westcott says.

Excuse: "I'm too old."

Reality: That's not what some iron-pumping octogenarians, nonagenarians, and even centenarians thought. Some of the most dramatic results of weight training have occurred in these people, says Dr. Westcott. "Older people who lift weights regain some of the strength of their youth and are able to function much better in life."

"If you work out regularly, you can be 50 and have a better body than a 25-year-old who doesn't work out," Andes adds.

Excuse: "I'll get huge muscles and look manly."

Reality: Most women don't have the time or testosterone to look like body builders. That takes enormous time—four to five hours per day—and the right genes, plus possibly steroids. "No one gets bulked up like that by accident," says Dr. Zelasko.

Besides, most adults have been losing muscle for at least 10 years. So any muscle you build is probably just replacing what used to be there. And muscle is actually more dense than fat, so it weighs more but takes up less space. In *Bone-Building Body-Shaping Workout*, author Joyce Vedral describes muscle as a silver dollar and fat as a sponge. The silver dollar weighs more, but the sponge takes up more space. So you may weigh a bit more when you build muscle, but the more of it you have, the slimmer you'll look.

Excuse: "I'll have to go to a gym."

Reality: "You can achieve a lot at home with free weights or band workouts," Andes says.

Still, gyms do have some advantages. They have a variety of resistance machines, which allow you to work your muscles in more ways, says Dr. Zelasko. There are also trainers available to teach you proper technique or show you how to use the equipment. Plus, the sight of other people working out can be inspiring.

Andes, who is not a fan of noisy, jam-packed health clubs, suggests some ways to come to peace with them: Wear a Walkman to block out other people, and go in the morning, when exercisers tend to be fewer.

Excuse: "I tried lifting weights before, but I didn't see any results."

Reality: The most common mistake that women make is using weights that are too light. "I see women at the gym lifting 2-pound weights that just aren't going to do anything for them," says Dr. Zelasko. "They're afraid they're going to get too big. But lifting a 10-pound weight won't give you huge muscles. Think about how many pounds you're maneuvering when you carry groceries or pick up a child. You're already lifting that kind of weight," he says. Muscles need to be subjected to more weight than they are used to in order for them to get stronger and more shapely.

Excuse: "If I stop exercising, my muscles will turn to fat."

Reality: "Muscles and fat are two different kinds of tissue; one can never be magically transformed into another," says Dr. Westcott.

"When I stopped for a few weeks, I was the same size, but I lost the definition in my muscles," adds exerciser deVries Ames.

The good news is that once you build muscles, they retain a kind of memory. They return quickly once you start to retrain them. "It's like riding a bicycle," says Cassandra Creech, an actress who lifts weights three or four times a week. "Once I get back to my routine after a layoff, my body knows just what to do."

Getting Started

Does a gym feel too daunting? Are you put off by rows of shiny machines? If that's the case, get expert advice. "You can learn the basic weight-training skills from a personal trainer in just two to five sessions," says J. P. Slovak, fitness director at the Cooper Fitness Center in Dallas. Although many people think of trainers as a prerogative of the rich, they're actually quite reasonable when you're interested in only a few sessions—only about $20 to $50 an hour. You'd pay that much for one night out on the town, for a hair appointment, or for a new pair of pants. Not a big sacrifice when you're talking about a new you.

A trainer will design a program for your specific needs, show you how to adjust the equipment, and simply give you the lay of the land. A trainer can also determine how much weight you need to lift to see results without getting injured. Once you've gotten started, "check in with the trainer periodically, say, every month, to evaluate your progress and fine-tune your routine," Slovak says. Just make sure that your trainer is certified by a reputable organization such as the American College of Sports Medicine, the Cooper Institute, the National Strength and Conditioning Association, or the American Council on Exercise (ACE). For an ACE-certified trainer in your area, call directory assistance for a toll-free number.

Keep It Going

Keeping records of your progress can help keep you going. Stacy Shishimabukuro, fitness manager of the Sports Club/LA in West Los Angeles, recommends that you get a buddy to take "before" measurements of your chest, waist, hips, thighs, calves, and arms. Then, update the figures every four to six weeks. "When you see that an inch has been taken off, it's really motivating," she says.

The process also can be intrinsically enjoyable. "I work out in the mornings; it's my hour of focusing," says Creech. "Weight training makes me feel powerful because I can control the changes in my body."

Adds deVries Ames, "When I don't work out, I feel sluggish, more depressed. But when I am in a good routine, I feel like I can do anything."

And in the end, it's the inner and outer results that count. "First, my posture got much better," says McCoy. "Then, I got a waist again. My arms got toned, and my derriere stopped drooping. I just couldn't wait for summer. It was so nice not to have to worry about camouflaging my body. I looked forward to showing it off."

How to Fall in Love with Exercise

When it comes to getting paired up, you know how elusive a suitable match can be. One relationship ends out of boredom, another from lack of commitment. Others just don't get your heart pounding. Or you don't even have time to think about it. Then you meet that special someone. It's fun. You're inseparable. You think, "This is the one." But six months later, polishing your silver looks more appealing.

Kind of sounds like your last workout program, right? Well, that's about to change. You're about to discover, for the first time, which workouts are "your type." In other words, which are really going to stick around this time. You know, till death do you part.

But you don't have to take out a personal ad to find "your type." Instead, try a personality test. They've been used for decades to counsel students toward the best career choices. Personality tests are also used to improve professional performance and business relationships and even such mundane activities as buying a car.

So why haven't you used one to find an exercise match? Because an exercise-oriented personality test didn't exist until now. Expert Charles Yokomoto, Ph.D., a consultant in Indianapolis who for years has studied personality type and sports, has created one.

Pairing exercise to your personality makes sense, Dr. Yokomoto says. Someone whose kitchen cupboards are organized alphabetically may fare best with a workout that has rules and parameters. Someone who prefers going standby for vacations will appreciate exercise that's more free-flowing. "When there's a mismatch, you're more likely to reject exercise without really knowing why," he adds.

Take the quiz, tally up your score, then read on to find out which kind of aerobic workout is most likely to guarantee you fitness success.

What's Your Workout Personality?

Following is a list of questions that may help you find a workout that you can stick with. Every question has four different descriptions that may or may not apply to you. Using the numbers 4 to 1, order these descriptions from the one that describes you most (4), to the one that describes you least (1). Remember, each description gets a number, and you can only use each number once per question.

Most like me	4
Somewhat like me	3
Hardly like me	2
Least like me	1

1. When contemplating my weekend activities, I prefer to:
___ a. Plan several days in advance.
___ b. Keep my options open until Friday.
___ c. Select activities that are intellectually stimulating.
___ d. Select activities that help my personal growth.

2. If I were a team leader, my style would be to:

____ a. Inspire people to develop their potential.

____ b. Resolve crises and conflicts after they arise.

____ c. Develop clear procedures and practices.

____ d. Study principles of good leadership and incorporate them into my leadership style.

3. If I could choose a particular office function to be in charge of, I would like to be responsible for:

____ a. Making the office a fun place to work.

____ b. Compiling a reading list of books that I felt people should read.

____ c. Developing personal-growth workshops for those who want them.

____ d. Developing a training guide that describes office procedures.

4. In relationships with others:

____ a. I am seen to be idealistic.

____ b. I am sometimes late for appointments because I get involved in something fun and forget the time.

____ c. I am known to get impatient when I'm not understood.

____ d. I often have expectations of how others should behave.

5. When I take part in activities such as games and sports:

____ a. I tend to play more on emotion and inspiration than strategies.

____ b. I tend to use conservative, conventional strategies that have been proven to be successful by others.

____ c. I like to create my own strategies.

____ d. I basically just try to have fun.

6. Those who know me well say:

____ a. I am empathetic and inspirational.

____ b. I am reliable and dependable.

____ c. I am intelligent and clever.

____ d. I am fun to have around when things become dull.

7. When it comes to taking part in planning activities at work or at home:

____ a. I like to see the big picture.

____ b. I like to get it done quickly and go on to something more enjoyable.

____ c. I like to inspire others to contribute their good ideas.

____ d. I like to be methodical and not miss any important details.

8. When a supervisor wants to compliment me for something done well:

____ a. I like to hear how cleverly I reacted to a crisis.

____ b. I usually already know.

____ c. I like to hear how valuable I am.

____ d. I like to hear how responsible I am.

9. When trying to resolve a problem at work or at home:

____ a. I am good at coming up with an intuitive solution.

____ b. I am patient with complicated problems.

____ c. I prefer tried-and-true solutions.

____ d. I tend to select a quick fix and not dwell on it.

10. If my close friends were to be honest, they would say that:

____ a. I tend to hold firm to my opinions.

____ b. I am flexible to the point that I change my mind a lot.

____ c. I am intellectually curious.

____ d. I am good at listening to problems.

Now transfer your answers to the table below. Notice that the spaces for scoring are not always in a–b–c–d order. After you've filled in all your answers, total your points in each column. The column with the highest number indicates your preferred workout style. If your two highest totals are nearly equal, it may mean that you're able to adapt well to both workout styles. Read the descriptions under both types to see which fits you best.

Example: b. 4   a. 2   c. 1   d. 3

1.	a.____	b.____	c.____	d.____
2.	c.____	b.____	d.____	a.____
3.	d.____	a.____	b.____	c.____
4.	d.____	b.____	c.____	a.____
5.	b.____	d.____	c.____	a.____
6.	b.____	d.____	c.____	a.____
7.	d.____	b.____	a.____	c.____
8.	d.____	a.____	b.____	c.____
9.	c.____	d.____	b.____	a.____
10.	a.____	b.____	c.____	d.____
TOTAL	a.____	b.____	c.____	d.____
	Organized	Spontaneous	Analytical	Inspirational

What Your Type Means

Organized

You feel best when life is orderly. In your home, there's a place for everything, and you like to keep it that way. You're punctual, dutiful, and once you agree to something, you're likely to follow through. You like rules and routine.

Your exercise Rx: Result-oriented workout. You like a schedule. It's no problem for you to set aside a block of time each day for exercise or even to stick with an activity that's repetitious. But to keep your interest, you need feedback. That's why cardio machines, which let you methodically monitor your progress, might be just the ticket. Most have computers that track your heart rate, calories burned, and distance traveled.

If you prefer the outdoor versions of repetitive sports, keep a fitness log to monitor your progress. And look for organized sports that will pose a challenge that you can prepare to meet. Signing up for a 5-K run/walk might be a good idea. Or set your sights on a mountain summit—and prepare for that challenge with a daily walk or run that steadily builds your endurance.

Best Choices for the Organized Personality

Treadmills	Walking
Stairclimbers	Cycling
Stationary bikes	Swimming
Running	

Spontaneous

Life is a game and your strategy is always changing. Doing the same thing over and over again is boring. You're good at handling crises, partly because you often find yourself in the middle of one of your own creation. But you're impatient with complex theories.

While you aren't much for rules, you'll follow them if they're simple and help you have fun.

Your exercise Rx: Short-but-sweet activities. Lifestyle activities that allow you to accumulate exercise time throughout the day may be a good choice, says Ross Andersen, Ph.D., director of exercise science at the Johns Hopkins weight management center in Baltimore.

Walk for 15 minutes after lunch, then for another 15 minutes after dinner. Park as far away from your destination as possible and expend energy taking the stairs. Ride your bike on the weekends or go for hikes. Spontaneous types also tend to do well with games. You'll probably find that you're naturally attracted to sports where you can join in any time. Join a softball or volleyball league, and you'll be in line for plenty of action. For a winter sport, skiing might suit you fine.

Best Choices for the Spontaneous Personality

Short walks throughout the day	Racquetball
Taking the stairs	Squash
Bike rides	Basketball
Hiking	Frisbee
Tennis	

Analytical

You don't mind complexity. In fact, you enjoy working out problems and puzzles and learning the theories and principles behind them. Your goal is to be competent at whatever you do. If an activity is too simple, you may drop out in search of something more challenging. You are also imaginative, but like things to make sense.

Your exercise Rx: Diversity training. Since analytical types fare best with a challenge and variety, cross-training may be the perfect option. You have the challenge of developing your own program, but keep potentially tedious activities fresh by mixing them up. Try a schedule that works something like this: Monday, 20 minutes on the stairclimber, 20 minutes on the stationary bike; Wednesday, aerobics class; Friday, 20 minutes on the cross-country ski machine, 20 minutes on the rowing machine. On alternate days, take up an activity that requires you to develop new skills.

You don't like to "do for the sake of doing." Instead, you appreciate why your heart rate should reach 120 beats a minute during aerobic exercise or which muscles you're stretching when you do a lunge. Read up on whatever activity you choose, to help keep your interest and improve your skills.

Someone with an analytical frame of mind often appreciates the "finer points" of a sport. Golf lends itself to this kind of personality, as you analyze your last stroke and think about your next one. Other good outdoor challenges are rock climbing, with all the technical difficulties it presents, and orienteering, a sport that calls for thoughtful deliberation.

Universal Exercise Barriers

Don't let these barriers to exercise that are common to all personality types stand in your way.

Time. Perceived lack of time is the biggest hurdle for exercisers, says Ross Andersen, Ph.D., director of exercise science at the Johns Hopkins weight management center in Baltimore. Notice that he said "perceived." You may have more time to exercise than you think. Make an appointment with yourself to exercise, and keep it just like you would any other appointment. If you have kids and feel that working out takes away from family time, make your family activities truly active: hike, take bike rides, or walk with your kids.

Going too slow or too fast. Besides choosing the fitness activity that's right for you, it's important to approach it at your own speed. "If it's not challenging enough, you'll get bored and drop out due to feelings of frustration," says Christina Frederick, Ph.D., assistant professor of psychology at Southern Utah University in Cedar City. "On the other hand, if it's overly challenging, you'll drop out."

If you're exercising alone, try adjusting the demands that you're making on yourself: Walk faster or vary your activities if you're bored, or slow down if the workout becomes uncomfortable. If you're taking a class that isn't keeping your interest, don't be afraid to switch instructors. "Some teachers are very good with a high-level class but can't

Best Choices for the Analytical Personality

Cross-training	Racquetball
Soccer	Squash
Tennis	Training for a triathlon
Sailing	

Inspirational

You're the type who catalyzes other people into action. You know how to say all the right things, which is why people gravitate toward you, tell you their problems, and look to you for inspiration. You're creative and are concerned about achieving personal growth.

Your exercise Rx: Dual-purpose exercise. To you, working out is engaging only when it's about more than just your body. You are more apt to enjoy it if it's about being part of a community—the reason why group

bring it down to beginners," points out Dr. Frederick.

Shyness. Admittedly, it's tough for everyone who wants to lose weight to put on exercise clothes and move her body in front of a bunch of strangers. But it may be particularly tough for people who feel shy and lonely. So tough, according to one study, that they may forgo exercising altogether.

"The gym can be intimidating, but people should realize that not all activities have to be done in a group," says study author Randy Page, Ph.D., professor of health education at the University of Idaho in Moscow. If you feel self-conscious about working out in front of others, try a home exercise machine or exercise video. Ultimately, it may even help you conquer your shyness. "As you become more physically active and feel better about yourself," theorizes Dr. Page, "you may end up feeling less shy."

Setting unrealistic goals. Having a goal of, say, exercising for one hour, six days a week, is certainly an admirable aspiration . . . but not if it's impossible to work so much working out into your busy schedule. If your fitness goals are unattainable, you'll be less likely to meet them and more likely to give up on exercising altogether. So keep your goals modest. You could even start just by vowing to walk for 15 minutes three days a week. Once you accomplish that goal, it can give you the confidence to set your sights a little higher.

social activities like exercise classes and team sports are a natural selection for you—or about exploring your inner self. The creative side of you can appreciate the elaborate movements required in dance classes and water aerobics. The spiritual side of you may like the body-mind aspects of martial arts, the meditative aspects of trail running, the serenity of swimming laps, or the simple, contemplative pleasures of taking nature walks. To enhance your spiritual side, try listening to music to set the mood for a peaceful workout.

Best Choices for the Inspirational Personality

Softball	Martial arts
Volleyball	Trail running
Soccer	Swimming
Dance classes	Tai chi
Water aerobics	

Personality-Specific Barriers

Different personalities don't just take to different activities—they have to contend with different obstacles, too. Here's what you might find in your path and how to get around it.

Organized. Since you like things to run smoothly, glitches perpetrated by others can trip you up. If, for instance, you decide to try out an exercise class but the teacher is disorganized and lackadaisical, you're likely to drop it like a hot potato. Solution: Stick with workouts that you control.

Spontaneous. Your biggest enemy is an idle mind. Even short workouts can turn torturous if there's nothing to occupy your brain. Solution: Watch TV or listen to music while exercising, or grab a workout partner to talk with.

Analytical. Even a varied routine can become, well, too routine for you. If there's no challenge to your exercise, you're likely to turn into a no-show. But there are bound to be times when even the most diversified exercise regimen will seem more simplistic than you like; it's inescapable. Solution: Make a list of your reasons for exercising—your motivators—and refer to it when the going gets tough; and when you push past those times, reward yourself.

Inspirational. Because you may often engage in activities that involve instructors or coaches, you run the risk of being turned off by corrections or criticism aimed at you or anyone else in your group. Solution: Remind yourself that the teacher/coach is only trying to help you; if that doesn't work, look for a class or team that focuses more on teamwork or a teacher or coach whose style you prefer.

Of course, personality isn't the only thing that determines how much you'll like a fitness regimen. If you're motivated enough, you'll override any kind of mismatch standing in your way, says Dr. Yokomoto. But most of us don't want to try so hard. And taking personality into account may make getting out of bed an hour earlier or forgoing your favorite sitcom for a workout a bit easier.

Make It a Habit

How much you like a workout is key to making exercise a lifelong habit. "The people who stick with exercise are those who enjoy it. They do it out of fun and interest and because it's a challenge," says Christina

Frederick, Ph.D., assistant professor of psychology at Southern Utah University in Cedar City. "And in the long run, they're going to continue exercising long after they lose 5 or 10 pounds."

Sage Advice

Are You Asking for Diabetes?

Want extra inspiration to shed the five pounds that glommed on to your waist over the winter? Try this: A huge study confirms that even a small upward move in the scale jacks up your risk for developing Type II (non–insulin–dependent) diabetes, a serious disease. By how much? Just a five-pound gain increases your risk for diabetes by 10 percent.

Beat High Blood Pressure

"The attitude of many patients is, 'My blood pressure is so bad, and I'm so overweight, that there's no point in trying to lose weight,' so they simply take pills," says Daniel W. Jones, M.D., director of the division of hypertension at the University of Mississippi Medical Center in Jackson. In fact, a recent study shows that nothing could be further from the truth. Just a little bit of weight loss can have a long-lasting effect on the medication needs of someone with high blood pressure.

Dr. Jones and his team found that, in a group of 102 volunteers with severe hypertension (high blood pressure), those who participated in a weight-loss program dropped an average of seven pounds after six months. This was enough to allow them to maintain healthy blood pressures with fewer drugs or smaller medication doses than the subjects who hadn't participated in the program's monthly classes and nutritional counseling.

Remarkably, this effect remained even after the people regained the weight they had lost. "The patients only maintained their weight loss for 6 to 12 months, but the benefits were sustained for as long as 30 months," Dr. Jones says. The reason why weight loss has such a prolonged impact on hypertension is unknown.

If cutting down on hypertension medication (and its cost and side effects) through weight loss appeals to you, ask your doctor if he'll monitor your blood pressure and cut your medication once you weigh less. "I think the vast majority of practitioners would be very receptive to that idea," Dr. Jones says.

Don't Wait to Ask about Weight-Loss Drugs

Call your doctor right now if you used the diet drugs Fen-phen or Redux before they were taken off the market and if you haven't been checked yet for signs of heart or lung disease. You probably know that fenfluramine (the "fen" in Fen-phen) and dexfenfluramine (trade name Redux) were pulled from the shelves, but you may not have heard that the Department of Health and Human Services has recommended that anyone who has used these drugs for any length of time get checked, particularly if you're planning any invasive medical or dental procedure. The drugs have been linked to a heart valve disease that can occur without any obvious symptoms. Your physician will know what to look for.

When You Can't Eat Just One

You're all alone with a bag of M&M's. Know how many you'll let yourself eat? It very much depends on how big that bag is, a study shows. When University of Illinois, Chicago, marketing professor Brian Wansink, Ph.D., gave people bags, containing 114 M&M's for a TV snack, they took an average of 63 pieces (a total of 209 calories). But given a bag with three times as many M&M's, people took an average of 103 M&M's (for a total of 341 calories). The bigger the stash of M&M's, the more M&M's people ate. The moral of this story is, if you're buying candy or any other high-cal temptation, buy small. Giant-size "economy" snacks make willpower go poof.

Hungry? Don't Blame Your Workout

Researchers aren't sure why people think exercise increases their appetites, but a review of studies on the topic says it isn't so. The results of more than 100 studies show that if you burn, say, 300 calories exercising, you won't compensate for them by eating more, especially if you're overweight. (Normal-weight folks do tend to compensate, which makes sense since their weight remains stable.)

One glitch, though, is that if you refuel with high-fat foods after a workout, you're likely to eat more calories than you burned, negating any weight-loss benefit, warns Angelo Tremblay, Ph.D., professor of physiology and nutrition at Laval University in Quebec and one of the study's authors. So after your walk, run, or ride, choose complex carbohydrates such as fruits, vegetables, and whole grains if you're hungry.

What Your Scale Isn't Telling You

Stop obsessing about the number on the scale—it doesn't tell you the whole story. Even more important than your weight is your percentage of body fat. It's fat, not necessarily the number on the scale, that puts you at increased risk for many diseases, says Steven Heymsfield, M.D., director of the weight control unit at the St. Luke's–Roosevelt Hospital in New York City. And the two don't correlate well.

The scale may tell you that you're overweight, but if a good portion of your weight is muscle, your percentage of body fat may be healthy. So there's no need to lose weight. And vice versa. The scale's number may look good, but if you're crash-dieting and not exercising, more of those pounds may be fat than muscle. But you'd only know that with a body composition test.

So how do you get one? Several options are available for home use. These are the three basic types.

Bioelectrical impedance (BIA). An electrical current is sent through your body—you don't feel a thing. How quickly it flows determines your body fat.

Skin-fold measurements. Pinch an inch (or more or less) at various sites on your body and then use a caliper to measure the folds.

Anthropometric measurements. They're the good ol' 36-26-36-type measurements. Using a tape measure, you record various body circumferences.

No matter which method you choose, here are some general guidelines for getting accurate measurements.

- Pick one method and stick with it. Measurements can vary among devices.
- Measure yourself monthly under similar conditions. Time of day, menstrual cycles, eating, and exercise can affect results.
- Don't get obsessed about another number. No method is 100 percent accurate, and each may vary up to 10 percent. Instead, focus on changes in the number. If it starts going up, but the number on the scale hasn't changed, you're losing muscle and replacing it with fat. Time to take action. If you're exercising and eating right, you should see the number go down.

Herbal Elixirs

Can You Lose with Herbal Supplements?

Herb expert and Prevention *advisor Varro E. Tyler, Ph.D., Sc.D., provides the skinny on today's most popular herbal diet pills.*

With the powerful prescription diet pills Redux (dexfenfluramine) and fenfluramine pulled off the market following reports of serious heart valve problems, many people are turning to natural, herbal alternatives. But natural doesn't necessarily mean free from side effects. Here's what Dr. Tyler has to say about the major herbal "quick fixes" in the marketplace.

HCA

What is it? HCA stands for hydroxycitric acid and is obtained from the fruit of *Garcinia cambogia*, commonly known as the brindall berry.

Where is it found? In products such as CitriMax and CitraLean.

Does it work? No good studies have demonstrated HCA's effectiveness in humans. But in animal studies, HCA appears to reduce food intake by reducing appetite. How HCA apparently diminishes appetite remains unclear.

Should I take it? Of all the weight-loss aids discussed, HCA holds the most promise, but important questions must be answered before it can be recommended: Is HCA still active once it's extracted, concentrated, converted into salt, and then marketed as a supplement? (We know that you wouldn't get the levels studied by just eating the fruit.) Is it absorbed by humans in supplement form? And will you regain the weight when you stop taking it, as with other diet aids? Are there any side effects, and how long can you take it?

Herbal Laxatives and Diuretics

What are they? Herbs that increase bathroom trips form the basis of many weight-loss products. Parsley, juniper, and dandelion leaves are diuretic herbs. Common laxative herbs include aloe, rhubarb root, buckthorn, cascara, and especially senna.

Where are they found? In products like Super Dieter's Tea, Trim-Maxx Tea, and Water Pill.

Do they work? These herbal laxatives are powerful stimulants that can cause significant loss of body fluid. The result? The number on your scale drops quickly. The reality? All you've lost is water, not fat, which you'll gain back as soon as you stop taking the laxatives. Furthermore, prolonged use promotes a so-called laxative habit in which your bowels become dependent on the substances in order to function. Other side effects include severe abdominal cramping and diarrhea.

Should I take them? The most serious concern about laxative-based herbal products is low potassium levels resulting from large losses of fluid. Over time, this deficiency can produce cardiac irregularities and even heart failure. In recent years, the Food and Drug Administration (FDA) has received many reports of adverse effects, including the deaths of four young women, in which dieter's teas containing these herbs may have been a contributing factor.

Ephedra

What is it? Ephedra, or ma huang (*Ephedra sinica*) is an herb that, particularly in combination with caffeine, has been touted as an appetite suppressant and metabolic stimulant.

Where is it found? In products like Super Diet Max, Herba Fuel, and Metabolift.

Does it work? There is considerable literature about its slimming effects, with some modestly good results.

But as a pharmacologist friend of mine quipped, "You're bound to lose weight on this combo; you're so hyper that the soup slops out of the spoon before it can reach your mouth." That may be a slight exaggeration, but the side effects of these products need no embellishment.

Should I take it? No. Some 800 adverse reactions, including 22 deaths and a number of serious cardiovascular and nervous system effects, such as heart attack, stroke, and seizures, have been attributed to the consumption of ephedra, often in combination with caffeine-containing herbs.

Other possible side effects of ephedra include increases in blood pressure, nervousness, heart palpitations, headaches, dizziness, skin flushing, sleeplessness, and vomiting. The FDA has proposed limitations on the use of ephedra, suggesting no more than 8 milligrams of ephedra alkaloids in a six-hour period, or 24 milligrams per day for no longer than seven days. This makes it useless as a diet aid.

Ephedra and St.-John's-Wort

What is it? The name of this herbal combination is a copycat of the very popular prescription diet-drug combo of phentermine and fenfluramine. But this "natural" version isn't the same: Like phentermine, ephedra is a stimulant, but unlike fenfluramine, St.-John's-wort (*Hypericum perforatum*) is an antidepressant and lacks any weight-loss properties.

Where is it found? In products like Diet-Phen and Herbal Phen-Fen.

Does it work? There have been no clinical studies to show that this combination will enhance weight loss.

Should I take it? According to the FDA recommendation, ephedra should not be used for more than seven days. And because these two herbs produce different responses in the central nervous system, there is simply no logical reason to combine them.

Miscellaneous Herbs

What are they? Ginger, red pepper, garlic, kelp, burdock, chickweed, marshmallow root, and alfalfa have all been hailed for weight loss.

Where are they found? Combined and with diuretics and laxatives.

Do they work? There is no evidence to suggest that these herbs will work.

Should I take them? Save your money. Instead, season your food with herbs. Dress up low-fat dishes with parsley, basil, turmeric, cilantro, or any other favorite herb or spice instead of butter, heavy sauces, or oils. They're practically calorie-free and they're bursting with flavor. Or sip a cup of chamomile or peppermint tea when you get an urge to eat. The liquid will fill you up, and the relaxation from a warm brew may calm stress-induced cravings.

Fiber, Nature's Weight-Loss Winner

Although not advertised as a weight-loss aid, dietary fiber is your best bet of the natural supplements.

What is it? Fiber is the part of various fruits, nuts, vegetables, beans, and whole grains that is not fully broken down in the digestive process.

Where is it found? In the foods listed above. If you're following a low-calorie diet or are unable to get enough fiber from food alone, supplements can help. Adding oat or barley bran, psyllium (in products such as Metamucil and Fibersol), or glucomannan capsules to your diet is an easy way to increase your fiber total.

Does it work? One study of 52 people found that those who dieted and also took a fiber supplement of seven grams a day lost nearly double the amount of weight of those who only dieted (12.1 pounds versus 6.6

pounds). The fiber group also said they were less hungry, while the others reported an increase in hunger.

Should I take it? Diets high in fiber ("high" is up to 35 grams a day) reduce the number of calories that the body absorbs from food by 30 to 180 calories daily, which over the course of a year could result in a loss of up to 19 pounds. A high-fiber diet can also help lower cholesterol, reduce the risk of colon cancer, and prevent or ease constipation.

To add fiber to your diet, start with small amounts and increase gradually to avoid diarrhea and flatulence. Follow label instructions and drink plenty of fluids with psyllium and glucomannan products because they can swell when ingested and cause throat obstructions.

Healing Moves

Tone and Shape Your Key Trouble Spots

Okay, so there's no such thing as spot-reducing. But you can firm up sagging muscles and straighten up your posture for a leaner look. Here's how-to advice from Miriam E. Nelson, Ph.D., associate chief of the physiology laboratory at the Jean Mayer U. S. Department of Agriculture Human Nutrition Research Center on Aging at Tufts University in Medford, Massachusetts, and author of *Strong Women Stay Slim* and the bestseller *Strong Women Stay Young*.

Keep in mind that as you progress in strength training, adding more exercises and heavier weights to your routine, it's important to warm up before you get started and to finish with some stretching. Don't worry: This won't keep you pumping iron throughout the entire Thursday-night lineup on TV. If you're already doing an aerobic workout, like walking, before lifting weights, you're warmed up. Otherwise, simply do a preset of each exercise with very light weights or none at all. This will get your blood pumping, warm up your muscles, and protect you from injury.

After a workout, take a few minutes to stretch the muscles that you just exercised. It's the best time to stretch, because your muscles are warm and more elastic. Only stretch as far as is comfortable. Hold each stretch for 20 to 30 seconds, concentrating on relaxing, breathing, and stretching the muscle. Don't bounce.

Coupling strength training with stretching increases not only the strength and tone of your muscles but also your flexibility. The resulting combination of strong muscles and flexibility helps prevent injury and keeps muscles in optimal condition as you age.

Note: If you experience persistent pain, ask a certified instructor at your local gym to teach you an alternate exercise. You may also want to see your doctor.

Look Five Pounds Thinner

Nothing makes you look more beautiful or slimmer than a strong back. You stand taller, look great in a bathing suit, and exude a great sense of self-confidence. In fact, adopting great posture and supporting it with a strong back can make you look at least five pounds lighter. To get a strong, shapely back, try this exercise, the bent-over row. It trains a host of back muscles: the latissimus dorsi (lats, for short), a large triangular-shaped muscle of the lower back that attaches to your upper arms; the trapezius, another large, kite-shaped muscle, which extends across the upper back; and the rhomboid muscles that lie underneath the trapezius. Plus, your biceps (in the upper arms) get a bonus workout.

When you're doing these lifts, take three seconds to raise the weight, pause for one second, then take a full three seconds to lower it again. Eight to 12 lifts are considered a set. Do one to three sets on each side. Do two to three sessions per week and allow at least one day of rest between workouts. And always remember to breathe evenly as you're doing the exercise—never holding your breath as you lift or lower the weight.

As you're trying this exercise, keep these very important pointers in mind: Don't rotate your torso as you lift. Don't look up; keep your neck straight, in a position parallel with your back. And your back should also be straight, not arched. Avoid scrunching your shoulders and neck, and make sure that you keep your supporting leg straight, not bent.

For best results, use a sturdy padded weight bench or piano bench to do the exercise. Or try using two armless chairs side by side.

Your back should be parallel to the floor. Let your arm hang straight down, and keep your shoulders even. The dumbbell should be directly under your shoulder and parallel to the floor. Keep your foot flat on the floor. Extend your leg, but don't lock it.

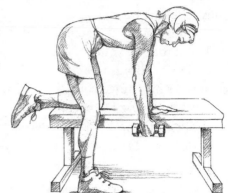

Pull the dumbbell straight up by bending your elbow. The dumbbell should remain parallel to the floor. Keep your elbow and the dumbbell close to your body.

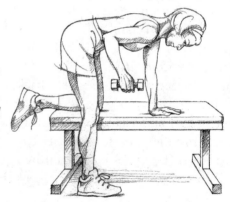

Continue until the dumbbell touches your ribcage and your elbow is slightly higher than your shoulder. Hold, then lower.

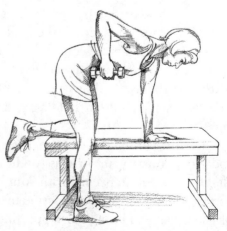

Trim Your Tummy

Okay, so you wouldn't be caught dead in one of those barely-there crop tops. That's still no excuse for letting your belly go to pot. In fact, it's more important for forty- and fifty-somethings to have strong, shapely abs than it is for the twenty-somethings sporting the crop tops: Strong abdominal muscles protect your back from injury. Along with your back muscles, your abs also help you maintain good posture, even as you get older. And standing up straight makes you instantly look slimmer.

You're probably intimately acquainted with the abdominal crunch, but it's still the best at-home choice for abs. Crunches are great for strengthening and toning. What they won't do is burn off the fat that may be hiding those muscles. If you really want to uncover your abs, you'll also need to do aerobic exercise like walking or jogging—and buy a crop top, of course.

Make Your Crunches Count

Forget the 100-crunches-a-day routine. When it comes to trimmer tummies, it's quality, not quantity, that counts. (That goes for all strength-training exercises.) If you find yourself hacking away at 50 or more crunches, chances are that your abs aren't getting the best workout.

Eight to 12 crunches are considered a set. Do one to three sets during each session, and two to three sessions per week, allowing at least one day of rest between workouts. Each crunch should last three seconds on the lift, with a three-second pause and three seconds to lower. And always remember to breathe.

If you can't do 8 repetitions, the effort is too much. Try the easier version, described below. When you can easily do 12 repetitions, the effort is too little. Move to the harder version.

Easier version: Place your hands on your thighs. As you roll up, move your hands up your thighs.

Harder version: Lightly place your hands behind your head, with your elbows pointing out to the sides. Don't pull on your neck or use your hands to lift.

To get the most out of your efforts, do crunches with your arms crossed over your chest.

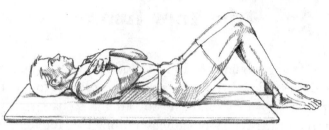

Bend your knees comfortably, at about a 90-degree angle. Place your feet about 12 inches apart. Tilt your pelvis so that your back is flat. Cross your arms over your chest. Focus your eyes on the ceiling.

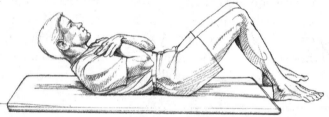

Using your abdominal muscles, lift your head and shoulders off the floor. Keep your neck and shoulders relaxed. Your lower back should always remain on the floor. As you roll up, slightly tip your chin toward your chest, but not too far. (Your fist should be able to fit between your chin and chest at all times.) Come up as far as is comfortable. Hold, and then lower yourself.

Keep your back straight, not arched, and move through the crunch slowly. Don't hook your feet or have someone hold them down; this minimizes abdominal effort. And don't come all the way up, or your hip flexors will do all the work.

Note: If you feel a strain in your neck, try relaxing it. If needed, lightly support your head with one hand. Just don't pull on your neck.

Shrink Your Hips

So there's a little extra jiggle on your hips these days. And it's tough getting back to center court after the crosscourt backhand. You need the side hip raise. It strengthens and tones the muscles on the outsides of your legs (hip abductors). These muscles are generally underworked and fairly weak. Build them, and you'll get agility, peak performance, and toned thighs and hips. And you might even get better balance. When combined with the leg-extension exercise, the side hip raise will help make your legs and hips very shapely.

Do one to three sets on each side, with 8 to 12 lifts in each set. Do two to three sessions per week and allow at least one day of rest between workouts. Each lift should last three seconds, with a one-second pause and three seconds to lower. And always remember to breathe regularly so you don't strain by holding your breath.

Do these exercises wearing ankle weights. If you can't do 8 repetitions, the weights are too heavy. When you can easily do 12 repetitions, the weights are too light.

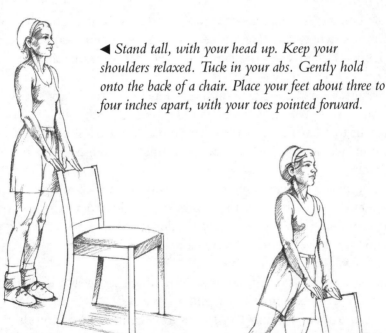

◀ *Stand tall, with your head up. Keep your shoulders relaxed. Tuck in your abs. Gently hold onto the back of a chair. Place your feet about three to four inches apart, with your toes pointed forward.*

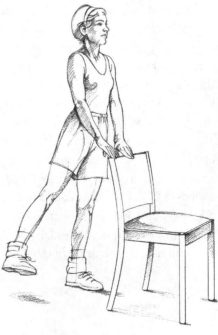

▶ *Slowly lift your right leg directly out to the side of your body, leading slightly with your heel. Keep your toes pointed forward and lift until your foot is 8 to 10 inches off the floor. Hold, then lower. Repeat with the other leg.*

Keep these important tips in mind as you're trying this exercise: Don't tilt your body to the opposite side as you raise your leg, and be sure to limit your lift to no more than 12 inches. Your feet should be pointed straight ahead as you're lifting, not to the sides or inward. And avoid gripping the back of the chair too tightly.

Build Leaner Legs

Your legs may be hiding under pants right now, but that's no reason to ignore them. Almost every move you make—walking, running, standing, climbing stairs—depends on your quadriceps, the muscles in the fronts of your thighs. They're not all work and no play, though. They put on the power when you ride a bike, climb a mountain, play tennis, or even pick up a child. Strong quads make every move easier and protect against injuries, especially ones to the knees.

This exercise, the leg extension, is the perfect exercise for strengthening your quads. You need a set of ankle weights, a sturdy chair (you'll need a chair that has a deep seat so that your knees are just off the edge), and a towel (add an extra towel under your thighs if your heels are touching the floor).

Each lift should last three seconds, with a one-second pause and three seconds to lower. Eight to 12 lifts are considered a set—and you should do one to three sets with each leg during each session. Do two to three sessions per week and allow at least one day of rest between workouts. And always remember to breathe.

If you can't do 8 repetitions, the weights are too heavy. When you can easily do 12 repetitions, the weights are too light.

There are several important things to keep in mind as you do this exercise: Don't sit with your knees more than two inches from the chair's edge. As you lift, don't lean back or arch your back. Also, be sure you don't move too quickly, and avoid lifting your thigh off the chair. And no fair gripping the chair to help you lift—that's cheating!

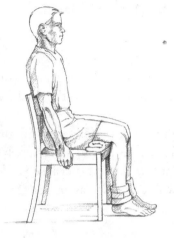

Keep your head up, with your eyes forward. Relax your arms at your sides. Sit back in the chair, keeping your back relaxed. Tuck in your abs. Put a rolled towel under your knees, making sure your knees are no more than two inches from the chair's edge. Place your feet shoulder-width apart; your heels should be just off the floor, with your toes lightly touching.

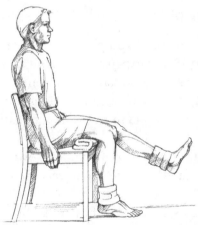

Slowly raise your left lower leg. The only joint that should be moving is the knee joint. Keep your ankle slightly flexed (toes pointing toward the ceiling). Continue lifting until your leg is fully extended.

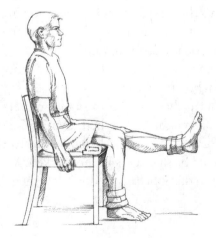

Hold, and then slowly lower your leg. Repeat with the other leg.

Build a Better-Looking Bustline

The best exercise for shaping and firming your bustline is the bench press, which targets the pectoral muscles in the chest. Plus, it sculpts your shoulders (the deltoid muscles) and tightens your triceps (the backs of your upper arms).

Besides flattering your figure, strong pectoral muscles can improve your tennis serve and golf swing. This exercise is similar to a pushup, but you don't have to get down on the floor to do it. And, because you're training three muscle groups at once, you will see results faster than if you just got single-muscle specific.

Equipment Info

You need a bench to do this exercise. If you plan to purchase one, all you need is the bare-bones variety. A less expensive option is an aerobic step bench. Or you may already have a good stand-in at home. Use a piano bench, picnic-table bench, or even a coffee table (as long as it has sturdy legs and doesn't have a glass top). Just add some padding to cushion your back.

For this exercise you'll need dumbbells—or, if you don't own a set, plastic gallon milk jugs with some sand or water. The recommended weight is five pounds.

Eight to 12 lifts are considered a set. Each lift should last three seconds, with a one-second pause and three seconds to lower. Do one to three sets in each session, and two to three sessions per week, allowing at least one day of rest between workouts. Again, remember to breathe as you're doing these exercises, so you don't end up straining.

If you can't do 8 repetitions, the weights are too heavy. When you can easily do 12 repetitions, the weights are too light.

When doing bench presses, keep these very important pointers in mind: Remember to keep your back straight, not arched. Don't raise the dumbbells back over your head, forward over your belly, or out to the sides of your body. Your elbows should be slightly bent, not locked. Move slowly when raising and lowering the dumbbells, and don't rest them on your chest.

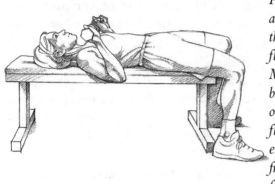

Lie on your back on the bench. Position the dumbbells about an inch above your chest. Keep the dumbbells parallel to the floor, palms facing forward. Make sure your head is on the bench, and straddle your legs over the bench. Keep your back flat on the bench. Point your elbows slightly down and away from your body. Keep your feet flat on the floor.

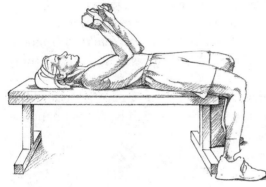

Slowly push the dumbbells straight up, away from your chest. The dumbbells should be about 18 inches apart and should remain parallel to the floor.

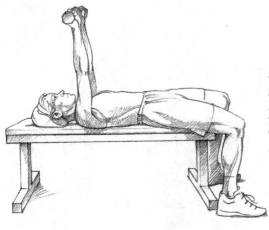

Fully extend your arms so that the dumbbells are directly above your chest. Hold, then slowly lower the dumbbells back down to the starting position.

Look Better from Behind

Glancing over your shoulder in a full-length mirror, you may notice a body part that's not immune to gravity: your derriere. But before you start trying to camouflage it in baggy pants, try this exercise, the hip extension, to strengthen and firm the gluteal muscles of your buttocks. (They're called glutes in gym-speak.) Even if you haven't seen signs of sagging, strong glutes will make bounding up stairs, standing, walking, and looking in the mirror easier. Combine this exercise with walking or other aerobic activities, and you'll like what you see behind you.

Each lift should last three seconds, with a one-second pause and three seconds to lower, breathing steadily all the time. Eight to 12 lifts are considered a set. Do one to three sets with each leg. Do two to three sessions per week, allowing at least one day of rest between workouts.

Do this exercise wearing ankle weights. If you can't do 8 repetitions, the weights are too heavy. When you can easily do 12 repetitions, the weights are too light.

As you're trying this exercise, keep these very important pointers in mind: Remember to grip the chair gently, not tightly. As you bend to-

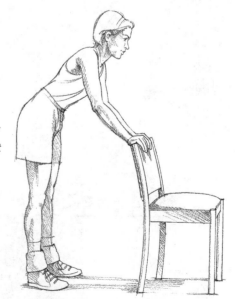

Stand about 12 to 18 inches behind a sturdy chair, gently holding on to it. Tuck in your abs and bend forward at the waist about 45 degrees. Align your head, neck, and back to form a straight line (check yourself in a mirror). Keep both legs straight, but don't lock your knees. Place your feet no more than shoulder-width apart, with your toes pointing forward.

ward the chair, don't let your upper body fall forward. Keep your toes straight, not pointed out to the side. And remember to lift your leg up and back, not out to the side.

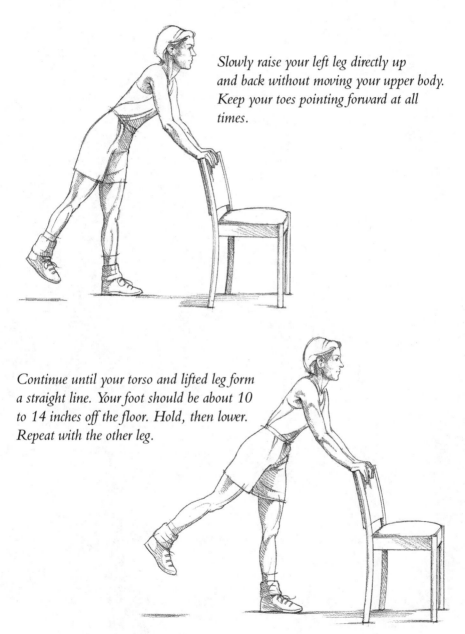

Slowly raise your left leg directly up and back without moving your upper body. Keep your toes pointing forward at all times.

Continue until your torso and lifted leg form a straight line. Your foot should be about 10 to 14 inches off the floor. Hold, then lower. Repeat with the other leg.

part

5

Feel
Your
Mental
Best

Making Sense of It All

A quick wit, a sharp mind, a photographic memory. Upbeat and optimistic. Inquisitive. Focused. High on energy yet in a state of quiet calm. The epitome of perfect mental health.

Most of us can only dream of feeling this good. But you can get closer than you ever imagined. No matter how old you are.

That's right, age is no barrier to improving your brainpower. And that may well be the best news of all. Failing memory, like weakening muscles, more often results from inactivity—or poor lifestyle habits—than from advancing age, as was once thought. Now, research tells us that keeping active mentally, as well as physically, can ensure us clear thinking and a positive outlook for life.

Are you ready to begin an exercise program for your brain?

In "Simple Ways to Sharpen Your Wits," you'll find mind stretches and brain calisthenics, of sorts, with proven benefit. The key is stimulation; don't retire from life. Your brain needs to be challenged, all the experts say. Read. Write. Travel. Learn a foreign language. Flex your mental muscles.

And how do you foster a sense of optimism and develop a healthy resilience to whatever comes your way?

Today's mantra is "Think young." Cultivate childlike qualities like playfulness, spontaneity, and joyousness. Here, leading psychologists will show you how. They'll tell you there's lots to be learned and gained from being a kid again.

Then, for relaxation of body and soul, try a little hands-on healing. Come along and discover the pleasures and lasting benefits of massage. You'll be amazed how this age-old natural remedy can melt away twentieth-century tension.

Finally, learn about the latest mind-body research involving diet, herbs, and exercise. The bottom line is, if you want to boost your brainpower, regularly top off your fruit, oatmeal, and fat-free milk with a multivitamin supplement and a brisk walk. And, for extra measure, try a little ginkgo—which may do wonders for your memory and for your sex life, too.

146

Positive Action Plans

Simple Ways to Sharpen Your Wits

Your brain is stupendous.

Okay, read those words again. Think how easily you understand each word—and all of them together.

Now, think about how you first learned to comprehend words. Years ago, you heard the word *your*, and it began to take on meaning. Later, you found out about *brain* and what it signifies—and that's something you've never forgotten. Later still, some teacher taught you how to read and pronounce *stupendous*, and you'll never have to look it up again.

That's just a small sampling of your nimble noggin at work. Multiply that kind of knowledge by millions, and you have a picture of your brain in action. In fact, in the powerhouse of your remarkable mind, you can store information equivalent to 20 million books the size of this one. A bookshelf holding all those books would be 631 miles long.

Not bad for a head that holds about three pounds of gray matter.

So how come the holding power of that incredible reservoir seems to start leaking at the seams as we age?

Maybe it's too full (20 million volumes of information is a lot to hold). Maybe all that intake of information gets a little—well—old, and we just don't pay attention as well as we used to.

Or maybe—and here's a radical thought—memory loss doesn't have to happen at all. Based on what researchers are discovering about the human brain and how it works, there's a good chance that you can actually protect your brainpower simply by using your mind more. And when you do that, you can actually protect yourself from aging.

"Your brain is the most important piece of real estate that you own," says Paul Spiers, Ph.D., a clinical neuropsychologist and visiting scientist at the Massachusetts Institute of Technology in Cambridge. "You need to do all necessary maintenance to keep it functional. You don't have to use a hammer and nails, of course, but you do need to keep your brain mentally and physically active to maintain its value."

If you've never thought of your brain as "active," maybe it's time to try some mental situps. Preserving or enhancing your brainpower doesn't mean that you have to take up ancient Greek or even recall pi to the 27th decimal place. It does mean that you might need to spend a few minutes every day putting that brain of yours through the equivalent of some calisthenics.

Keeping Your Mind Vigorous

The vast majority of us can maintain or even improve our mental vigor throughout our lives, according to K. Warner Schaie, Ph.D., director of the Gerontology Center at Pennsylvania State University in University Park. Maintaining a good diet and getting regular exercise can have a direct effect on the mind's ability to stay young, he notes. Many of the "natural" changes that are thought to occur with aging don't have to happen at all.

And if you want to put the mental brakes on aging, you need to regularly expose yourself to a wide range of mental challenges, from learning a new language or doing puzzles to writing, painting, or making music, according to Vernon Mark, M.D., a Newport, Rhode Island, neurologist and co-author of *Reversing Memory Loss*.

"There are people over 100 years old who are functioning very well mentally," Dr. Mark says. "One of the reasons for this is that they don't retire from life. They keep challenging themselves in new ways. That's important because the brain abhors boredom. You need to keep it stimulated."

Leo Tolstoy, famed Russian novelist, had his first bicycle lesson when he was 67. Queen Victoria started learning the Hindustani language when she was 68. Grandma Moses didn't begin painting until she was in her seventies.

At any age, new and challenging activities are the brain's best friend. "The most important ingredient for the brain is intellectual stimulation," Dr. Spiers says. "The more you can keep your brain doing things—reading, writing, traveling, learning new information—the more resistant your brain will be to the effects of aging."

Even doing familiar tasks can enrich your mind—if you add new twists. "If you're right-handed and try to play tennis with your left hand, then you're using a totally different set of reflexes," says Arnold Scheibel, M.D., professor of neurobiology and psychiatry and former director of the Brain Research Institute at the University of California, Los Angeles. "Everything that you're doing is essentially reversed, and that makes it the equivalent of a totally new experience."

Brain Pleasers

The important point is that you don't have to take on enormously difficult challenges to make substantial improvements in how well your brain works. Doing anything new or different will help strengthen your brain and keep your mind sharp. Here are some tips that experts recommend when you're adding rooms to your mental mansion.

Tease your brain at the market. Here's an easy way to flex your mental muscles. The next time you go shopping, leave the list in the car, says Michael Chafetz, Ph.D., a clinical psychologist in New Orleans and author of *Smart for Life*. Take a minute to memorize six or eight items that you need.

Once you're in the store, get a cart and pick a starting point. Go get your first item, then return to the starting point. Then get the rest of the items, one at a time, returning to the starting point each time.

That's all. This simple exercise will help strengthen your memory while at the same time improving your mind's ability to create a mental map of where things are, says Dr. Chafetz. When you do this regularly, you'll find that you can remember more and more things—not only groceries but also tasks that you need to do at work or home—at one time.

Turn off the telly. It's no accident that television became known as the boob tube. Researchers at Kansas State University in Manhattan, Kansas, found that people who watched just 15 minutes of television had diminished brain-wave activity, an indication that their minds were turning off. "For the most part, the images on that screen just flow through you without enhancing your life," Dr. Chafetz says.

He recommends making at least one night a week a no-television night. You may be surprised at the number of mind-stimulating alternatives that you'll come up with to fill the time.

Test with the tube. Although television is by nature a passive activity, there are ways to watch and still be mentally active, says Thomas Crook, Ph.D., director of Memory Assessment Clinics in Scottsdale, Arizona, and author of *How to Remember Names*. When watching TV, he says, jot down a few notes about facial expressions, clothing, or anything else that's happening on the screen. Set the notes aside. A day or two later, see how much you can recall. It's fun to put your memory to the test, and doing this for even a few minutes will help keep both your memory and powers of observation sharp, Dr. Crook says.

Tune in to pulp fiction. Why not pick up the latest bestseller and lose yourself in a thriller, mystery, or romance? Reading is a time-tested brain booster that helps improve language skills while keeping your memory strong, according to Dr. Chafetz.

You don't have to read Plato's *Republic* or Shakespeare's sonnets to exercise your mind. Even light reading can powerfully improve your word skills, says Dr. Chafetz. He recommends picking up a book or magazine daily and reading for at least 15 minutes.

Keep doing head counts. It wasn't so many years ago that most of us did math in our heads. These days, many clerks have a hard time making change unless the computer or calculator is telling them what to do. "If you use a calculator every time you have to add three numbers together, your mental abilities are going to suffer," Dr. Crook says.

Inscribe your thoughts. Few things clarify thoughts and improve memory and logic as well as writing does, says Alan S. Brown, Ph.D., professor of psychology at Southern Methodist University in Dallas and author of *How to Increase Your Memory Power*. Even if you don't fancy yourself a wordsmith, take a few minutes to write at least one letter a week to a friend or relative, he suggests. Or write a letter to the editor or a note evaluating a product that you recently bought. Anytime you pick up a pen instead of the telephone, you help keep your mind sharp, says Dr. Brown.

Create a challenge. Put your mind to work with a simple puzzle you can make at home, like the one that Dr. Mark suggests below. The larger, the better—and if you want to repeat the puzzle, make some photocopies. Any set of random numbers and letters will do the trick, says Dr. Mark. The goal is to circle in pencil certain numbers and letters within a given time. For instance, try to circle every "2" and every "c" within 15 seconds.

```
k 3 f g 8 4 g 3 c s 0 1 n z d 8 2 f g h 6 0 1
j l 5 d 9 v b 7 3 3 2 a b 6 c n 4 b q d 3 4 4 d
p u 6 v 9 1 u 8 v a 0 m n 2 h g z w 6 r y t 7
c 11 e c b q p b 9 7 m 3 6 g u w 3 c 2 3 8 u
2 4 h t y l 5 3 8 n e a 9 2 9 k m z 7 y 3 m 9
p h 4 f d s a 3 2 8 v m r 0 4 b 6 11 c d l 8
```

Repeat the exercise again on a fresh copy, finding a different set of numbers and letters. Doing this once or twice a week is a good way to help improve your concentration and attention span, Dr. Mark says.

Tie up your tongue. Doing tongue twisters not only improves speech but also helps improve concentration by exercising speech and language circuits , Dr. Chafetz says. At least once a day, he says, take a minute to practice your favorite tongue twister, like "fresh fried fish don't flip like fresh fish flip" five times in a row.

Be punny. Puns and other types of humor spark creativity and encourage your mind to look at problems in new ways, Dr. Chafetz says. Take a moment to really think about words you hear, and then see what odd twists you can come up with. For example, the word "illegal"—a sick eagle.

Cut it out. Take a few minutes to clip funny cartoons, photos, and stories from newspapers and magazines and put them up in your "humor gallery" in your home or office. Whether you're making your own humor or enjoying someone else's, you need to look at the world from odd angles. This change in perspective will help keep your mind active, Dr. Chafetz says.

Get cross with words. What's a five-letter word for "cowboys and Indians." Could be "fight" or "movie"—or maybe it's "teams"—as in the Dallas Cowboys and the Cleveland Indians.

With clues like that, crossword puzzles are a great way to puzzle your mind. And embracing their twisted logic may be one of the best things you can do for your brain. Doing crosswords and other puzzles exercises the brain cells involved in word retrieval, vocabulary, and comprehension, says Dr. Chafetz.

Add challenge to games. Chess, Scrabble, jigsaw puzzles, and other mind-stretching games are terrific challenges that help keep your mind clicking at a youthful tempo. But why not go a step further and give your brain an even tougher workout?

There are many ways to put a new twist on old games, says Dr. Chafetz. When playing Scrabble, for example, use some new rules. You can require that each word have a minimum number of letters, or you can limit the allowable words to nouns or adjectives. When doing a jigsaw puzzle, try turning it over and putting it together from the blank side.

And for chess aficionados, here's what Dr. Chafetz suggests to reach the height of mental challenge: Pick a worthy opponent, and blindfold

Aerobics to Step Up Your Brainpower

The mind-body connection isn't a one-way street. Just as your thoughts and emotions play a role in how your body feels, how you treat your body clearly affects your mind, says Barry Gordon, M.D., Ph.D., a neurologist at the Johns Hopkins Medical Institutions in Baltimore and author of *Memory: Remembering and Forgetting in Everyday Life*.

Research has shown, in fact, that regular exercise isn't just good for your heart and lungs. It can also pump up your brain power. In one study, researchers at Ohio State University in Columbus found that people who rode stationary bicycles three times a week for nine months were able to improve their attention span, concentration, and short-term memory. Other studies have shown that people who are active tend to have faster reflexes and think more quickly than those who aren't.

It doesn't take a lot of exercise to get the benefits, Dr. Gordon says. Simply doing some type of aerobic exercise, like walking, running, or swimming, for 20 minutes three times a week can make a significant difference.

yourself. Ask your opponent to call out the moves. See how long you can continue the game, just picturing the board in your mind. When you attempt this, you'll stimulate your imagination, focus your concentration, and put your logical skills to the test, says Dr. Chafetz.

Just imagine your braininess. With a technique called mental imagery—which you practice in bed, in the shower, or while standing in line at the store—you can readily improve your memory and powers of thinking, says Dennis Gersten, M.D., a San Diego psychiatrist and author of *Are You Getting Enlightened or Losing Your Mind?*

One of the simplest forms of mental imagery involves focusing on an image or situation, then using your imagination to embellish it with as much detail as you possibly can.

Here's an exercise you may want to try. Picture a cube in your mind. Imagine that each side is a different color. "There's a lot of mental effort involved in picturing a cube and consciously trying to rotate it," Dr. Gersten says. "You're really forcing your mind to work in a very active way."

In your mind, turn the cube from side to side, memorizing the colors as they appear. Then, rotate the cube again and predict the colors before they appear.

With a little practice, says Dr. Gersten, you'll soon find that it's easy to predict which colors will appear next. To make it a little more difficult, add more sides to the mental cube so it assumes another shape. You'll find that doing this simple exercise for five minutes twice a day will substantially improve your memory and help you think more clearly—not just while doing the exercise, but in all aspects of your life, he says.

Arts and the Craft of Mind Sharpening

Other favors that you can do for your wits and memory may take longer, but they're worth trying for lots of reasons. You may even find talents that you never knew you had. And the only risk is that you might enjoy yourself so much, you'll never want to give up what you've started.

Take up an instrument. Playing music brings an enormous number of skills into play, from improving coordination and concentration to fostering your creative instincts. And you don't have to practice six hours a day to get the benefits. Playing an instrument for 10 to 15 minutes a day will give your brain a good workout, Dr. Scheibel says.

Share your passion. From photography and pottery to Swedish and Swahili, we all have skills that we can share with others—and the challenge of teaching those skills is very good for the mind, says Dr. Brown. It's not hard to find a classroom to teach in, he adds. Most community centers and civic organizations are eager for volunteers who can teach hobbies, languages, or other skills.

Do anything classy. Perhaps you're more comfortable being in the class rather than in front of it. Adult education—be it Spanish, accounting, calligraphy, dancing—provides an excellent mental workout, Dr. Brown says. You'll discover stimulating ideas and people to discuss them with. Plus, studying for tests is a superb way to help improve your memory.

Being Upbeat

You are what you think. And if you happen to be a pessimist, researchers say, thinking can be dangerous to your wits.

"It has long been known that people behave a lot in terms of their self-perceptions," Dr. Schaie says. "Optimists tend to get involved in activities that stretch them, while pessimists may opt out and say, 'It's no use.' And if you stop doing things, your mental skills will eventually decline. It becomes a self-fulfilling prophecy."

When you're struggling with work, raising a family, and making enough money to pay the bills, it's not always easy to maintain an optimistic point of view. That's why Dr. Chafetz recommends that you keep a journal in which you jot down at least 20 good things that happen to you each day. Even small things, like finding a dollar under the sofa, count. Doing this regularly will help you feel more positive about yourself and life in general. This in turn will make you more likely to take on new challenges, keeping your brain active, Dr. Chafetz says.

It's also a good idea to push yourself in new directions, even if that means occasionally failing, says Jack Matson, Ph.D., director of the Leonard Innovation Center at Pennsylvania State University in University Park. "Taking a risk increases your passion because you've put your soul out there for all to see. Even if you fail, it generally forces you to think more deeply about the problem and brainstorm other possible ways to solve it."

Cultivate the Child inside You

Poised at the edge of a 225-foot drop-off, Gary Kyriazi smiles and leans back in his seat.

Suddenly, the seat lurches forward, and plummets.

And Kyriazi howls with delight. "Whoooooooooooooooaaaaaahhh!"

A passenger on the Desperado, a gigantic steel roller coaster in State Line, Nevada, Kyriazi is whisked down, through a hole in the ground, back to Earth's surface, then in and out of a series of rapid rises and drops that leave him momentarily airborne.

A roller coaster fanatic, Kyriazi, 47, has been on the Desperado plenty of times before. He has been on numerous other coasters, too. But every ride is a thrill, he says.

"I like the speed, the freedom, the feeling of flight—it's an incredibly fun experience," says Kyriazi, who works as an independent consultant for the amusement industry in New River, Arizona, and happily drives four hours north to State Line for an 80-mile-per-hour spin on the Desperado.

The author of *The Great American Amusement Parks*, Kyriazi has been riding roller coasters since he was two years old. (His first fling was on a pint-sized kiddie coaster.) He rides as often as possible.

"Riding roller coasters makes me feel happy," says Kyriazi. "By nature, I'm young at heart. Riding roller coasters is a way of expressing it, and it's part of my job."

Coast Back to Childlike

The truth is, riding roller coasters can help *you* stay young at heart, too. So can reveling in all sorts of other experiences that cultivate childlike qualities—like playfulness, spontaneity, joyousness, flexibility, and optimism.

It's a worthwhile investment of time and energy. Why? These kidlike qualities confer substantial benefits. Studies find that people who are optimistic and playful live longer, healthier, and happier lives.

"We're not talking about being child*ish*," says Joel Goodman, Ed.D., director of The Humor Project in Saratoga Springs, New York. "It's important to distinguish between being child*like*—being spontaneous and flexible and so forth—and being child*ish*. Being childish is being irresponsible and immature. But being childlike can be a very mature way of coping with and enjoying life."

But what if you weren't particularly spontaneous or flexible as a kid? Well, you can still cultivate these kidlike qualities as an adult. It's just a matter of knowing how.

One of the benefits of growing up and becoming an adult is that you can change, says Bonnie Jacobson, Ph.D., a clinical psychologist and director of the New York Institute for Psychological Change in New York City and author of *If Only You Would Listen*. You can cultivate these qualities now even if you didn't have them then.

"When you're a child, you just are, but when you're an adult, you have the ability to choose how you want to be," says Dr. Jacobson. "You can develop strategies to change."

Ready, Set, Revel

This very moment, you can start making the kind of changes that cultivate kidlike qualities. All you have to do is revel in assorted kidlike pleasures. So get ready, get set, and . . .

Laugh your head off. A sense of humor offers bona fide age-protecting benefits. Studies suggest that it can both improve the quality of, and lengthen, your life. Among other things, humor seems to help insulate you from stress. In a series of studies, women executives who scored high on tests designed to measure sense of humor felt less stressed out, had fewer stress-related health problems, were less likely to get burned out, and had higher self-esteem than those who scored low.

In other studies, humor has been shown to improve problem solving and creativity. And humor often goes hand in hand with other age-protecting attributes like resilience, says Irene Deitch, Ph.D., professor of psychology and chairwoman of Options, a college study program for older adults, at the College of Staten Island in New York City.

"People who are resilient often have a good sense of humor," says Dr. Deitch. "When the going gets tough, they use humor to cope."

Play for the sake of playing. Before adults teach them to "play to win," most kids play simply to have fun.

"Children take pleasure in playing for the sake of playing," says Carolyn Saarni, Ph.D., developmental psychologist and professor in the graduate department of counseling at Sonoma State University in Rohnert Park, California. "They do it for the sensory and experiential value; they don't have to achieve and win all the time."

Unfortunately, many of us grow less playful and more preoccupied with winning as we grow older. To reclaim that playfulness that you enjoyed as a kid, Dr. Saarni suggests trying some new recreational pursuit.

"Learn to do something sensory and enjoyable—just for the sake of doing it, not so you can excel at it," she says. "When I was in my midforties, I decided to learn to scuba dive. I decided that I wasn't going to push myself, but simply enjoy the process of doing it. And it gives me great pleasure."

Go exploring. A psychologist in Chicago, Jonathan Smith, Ph.D., has spent more than a decade studying what he calls R-states. The "R" stands for relaxation, Dr. Smith explains. Aptly so, since R-states are characterized by feeling physically limp, distant, and at ease. When you're experiencing R-states, you also have feelings like optimism, hope, joy, and awe.

"R-states can rejuvenate and renew us," says Dr. Smith, founder and director of the Roosevelt University Stress Institute and professor of psychology at Roosevelt University in Chicago.

While kids seem to experience awe fairly regularly—in the course of discovering seemingly mundane things like birds' nests—we adults experience it less often, says Dan Gottlieb, Ph.D., a family therapist in Cherry Hill, New Jersey, and author of *Family Matters*.

If that weren't bad enough, some of us get less optimistic and less hopeful as we grow older, says Christopher Peterson, Ph.D., a professor of psychology at the University of Michigan at Ann Arbor.

But we can recapture those special feelings and experience R-states, Dr. Smith says. For example, first do something relaxing, he advises. Then do something simple and fun. "I'd say that being young at heart means being able to cultivate and savor R-states," he observes. To get in the right frame of mind to get into an R-state, you have to relax first, says Dr. Smith. A number of powerful relaxation techniques—including massage by a professional therapist—are good for cultivating different R-states. A professional massage might make you feel physically relaxed and calm, while yoga might make you feel refreshed and awake. And meditation may make you feel prayerful and spiritual. All of these techniques can help still your mind and prepare you for an R-state. Then, follow up with the simple and pleasurable activity of your choice, Dr. Smith says. If you don't want to explore the woods, try gardening, or go for a bike ride.

Take a nap. If you've been working on your taxes for two hours straight, take a break. Take a nap. Or take a walk around the block.

"Do any of those little things that give you immediate pleasure. You're entitled to a 10-minute snooze," says Dr. Saarni. "You'll feel better. You'll feel rejuvenated."

Get curiouser and curiouser. Ever notice how many questions kids ask? Did you? Ever? Huh?

Kids are full of curiosity, another of those attributes that makes life more vibrant.

"The payoff of curiosity is that your world becomes bigger," Dr. Saarni says. "If you're curious, your horizon keeps getting pushed back."

When we grow up, many of us grow less willing to ask questions, to try things that we don't know how to do. We worry that our questions will be "dumb." We think that we should already be expert in everything.

Again, the solution is to try something new and tell yourself that it's okay to be a novice, says Dr. Saarni. Then jump in and get wet behind the ears. Tune in to a radio call-in show and ask some questions. Sign up for that wine-tasting class at the local vineyard.

If you're a hard-driving type who finds the novice role terrifying, remind yourself that the alternative to being curious is being bored. "Tell yourself, 'If I don't try out new things, I'll have a very small little world,'" suggests Dr. Saarni.

Indulge in fantasy. When it comes to health and well-being, optimism is optimal. Research finds that people who score high on tests of optimism find greater pleasure in life, feel less hassled and stressed by everyday demands, report fewer health problems, even recover more quickly from major surgery, than those who get low scores.

You don't have to be a dreamer to be an optimist, but it helps, says Dr. Jacobson. One way to cultivate optimism is to pay attention to your daydreams and fantasies. But not all daydreams are created equal. "Either we're having positive fantasies or negative ones," she says. Tuning in to images of yourself winning the monthly sales award or finishing a 25-K race can brighten your outlook.

Surprisingly, you can also reap some benefits by tuning in to negative fantasies as well, according to Dr. Jacobson. If you really start paying attention to your negative fantasies—rather than letting them drone along in the background of your consciousness like a television that someone has forgotten to shut off—you'll start to see the flaws in them, he says.

"Eventually, negative fantasies begin to seem ridiculous to you," Dr. Jacobson says. "You get tired of them. And, automatically, they start to change."

Listen to your buddies. Chances are, you had a best friend when you were a kid. You were inseparable and told each other everything.

That kind of sharing is essential to forming and keeping close friendships, says Dr. Jacobson. Close relationships foster emotional health and contribute to physical well-being, as well. Various studies find that people with close relationships report greater satisfaction in life. If your close friends are optimistic and fun-loving all the better. Friends like these make us more resilient, says Dr. Jacobson.

To make close friends, you have to spend time listening to people talk, especially about themselves, she says. The more you let another person talk about himself, the more likely it is that you'll find common ground, the basis for close friendships.

Many of us don't put in enough time listening to one another, so our conversations linger on a fairly superficial level, as do our friendships, Dr. Jacobson says.

"If you're talking to someone you'd like to get close to, and they tell you that they were just in Rome and loved it, let them talk a long time about Rome," she suggests. "Let them talk long enough that you really get a sense of what they liked so much, so you really have something to talk about."

And practice what's known as active listening, says Marlene F. Watson, Ph.D., a couple and family therapist and director of graduate programs in couple and family therapy at Allegheny University of the Health Sciences in Philadelphia. After the other person has finished speaking, paraphrase what he has just said. This reassures the other person that you're really listening. And it gives you a chance to clear up any misunderstandings that might arise.

Long-Term Investments

Some kidlike pleasures make you feel young at heart right away. Others pay dividends after a longer investment. Here's how to invest your time and energy for maximum age-protecting results.

Remember the Boy Scout creed. Particularly the part about being trustworthy.

Life's rough spots can wear away trust and leave us cynical. And that's truly unfortunate. Living is a lot more stressful and less enjoyable when you don't trust. Not surprisingly, studies find that cynics have significantly more health problems than trusting types.

The thing about trust, though, is that you have to be trustworthy if you're going to trust others, says Dr. Saarni. "Trust is paradoxical," she says. "The way to rebuild trust in others is to put yourself in a position where people trust you."

If you're more cynical than you'd like to be, consider volunteering at a local school or respite center for mentally disabled adults, she suggests. "Mentally disabled folks tend to be trusting and inspire trust," Dr. Saarni says.

Savor your successes. Teach a five-year-old the lyrics to "Old MacDonald," and she'll happily croon it until the cows come home. Kids get a lot of satisfaction from everyday accomplishments. And that's a good thing since savoring your successes builds optimism, says Dr. Peterson.

"If you want to be more optimistic, one of the things you can do is define success in terms of things you can achieve," he says. "If you define success in such a way that you'll only feel successful if you earn a million dollars a year, you're setting yourself up for disappointment. If you tell yourself that you'll be a success if you can enjoy your work and put food on the table, you'll feel better about life and feel more optimistic."

Optimism is often self-fulfilling. Deriving satisfaction from one task can help you succeed at the next. "Research suggests that optimists are more successful at school and at work and tend to have more and better relationships," he adds. It only make sense. Because optimists expect things to work out eventually, they're persistent. Because they're persistent, things work out for them.

Make new friends. It's tough to be the new kid in town. And it's not much easier to be the new adult. But it happens. A lot. According to the Census Bureau, the average American moves 11 times in a lifetime.

In a culture this mobile, it helps to know how to make new friends. Spend some time watching kids play together, and you'll pick up some pointers, says Dr. Saarni.

"Watch kids who successfully negotiate what we call peer entry, and you'll see that they all do certain things," says Dr. Saarni. "These kids observe what's going on and try to join in the activity. They don't try to draw attention to themselves or try to take control or be in charge. They don't go up to other kids on the slide and say, 'Look, let me show you the best way to go down that slide.' If they did, they'd be rejected."

If you want to make new friends, your best bet is to join a group that's doing something you like. Love gardening? Go to a garden-club meeting. When you get there, look around, see what everyone else is doing, and join in. If the group is repotting mums for the upcoming plant sale, do the same. Whatever you do, don't be bossy, try to take control, or hog all the attention.

Forgive the bullies. If you spend time watching kids, especially little kids, you'll also pick up pointers on cultivating another talent—forgiving. "Forgiveness seems to be easier for children," says Gerald G. Jampolksy, M.D., a child and adult psychiatrist and the founder of the Center for Attitudinal Healing in Sausalito, California. "A five-year-old can get into a fight with a friend who has taken one of his toys and, five minutes later, forgive his friend and start playing with her again. But when adults fight, they may not speak to each other for years."

What happens? As we get bigger, so do our egos, says Dr. Jampolsky. We become more judgmental. "The more judgments we make, the more unforgiving we are, and the stronger the ego feels," he explains.

Unfortunately, though, there's a trade-off. Withholding forgiveness inflates your ego but undermines your peace of mind. Ironically, by refusing to forgive someone, you actually give that person considerable power over you and your well-being, he says.

But how can you really forgive someone who's done you wrong?

Assume the person is afraid, Dr. Jampolsky says. It's a safe assumption since most wrong-doing stems from fear. Consider the colleague who took credit for your idea for the Waldenstein account. Odds are, he did it out of fear of not looking good. Once you realize that he's afraid, it's easier to feel some compassion for the guy.

Keep in mind that forgiving doesn't mean condoning. You don't have to convince yourself that it was okay for your office mate to steal your idea. And you don't have to continue sharing your ideas with him. In fact, you may be better off if you don't. But if you remind yourself that he probably filched your idea out of fear, eventually, you can sympathize, forgive, and feel better. Research finds that forgiveness is often followed by a let-up in anger, depression, anxiety, and related emotions.

Plan for surprises. When you have to juggle multiple obligations—job, relationships, car maintenance—you have to schedule your time. Schedule every moment, though, and there's too little room for discovery or surprise.

Kids tend to have an innate appreciation for spontaneity, says Dr. Gottlieb. Not surprisingly, they have a knack for discovering all sorts of surprises, even amidst the ordinary, he says.

"One afternoon, I had a young friend, a three-year-old, dropped off at my house," Dr. Gottlieb recalls. "I'd been working frantically on about four different projects, like we all do. When she arrived, I said, 'What shall we do this afternoon?' And she said 'I don't know.' Anytime I asked her a question that had a time reference, she gave me a curt answer. So I decided that she, I, and the dog would go for a walk. Well, along the way she found an anthill, and she pulled me over to see it, and we watched that anthill for about 20 minutes. It was fascinating. We gave each of the ants a name and a role. And we talked about all sorts of ideas and feelings. We had a wonderful time."

Get creative. Give a kid a crayon, and he won't waste time berating his erstwhile muse or worrying what the critics will think. He'll color.

Kids are a lot less likely to edit their creative urges than we adults are, says Carolyn Adams-Price, Ph.D., associate professor of psychology and chair woman of the gerontology program at Mississippi State University in Starkville and author of *Creativity and Successful Aging*.

We adults, however, tend to have a lot more creative potential than kids do. "I'd say that creativity is being able to produce something that is meaningful or inspiring, something that other people can relate to or attach meaning to," Dr. Adams-Price says. "And adults are better able to do that."

If you've concluded that you're not creative because you didn't do well in art class, think again. There are innumerable ways to be creative—and most of us have talent for at least some of them, says Dr. Adams-Price. So try your hand at quilting, photography, papier-mâché, or sculpting with odd bits of wire and other found objects.

Recent research suggests that creative expression fosters openness, flexibility, playfulness, humor, and resilience—all boons to mental health.

Tell tales. As any teacher who has ever inquired about the whereabouts of a missing homework assignment can tell you, kids are good at telling stories. Not just when they have to, either. Kids make up stories for the sheer pleasure of telling them.

Storytelling is just one more way of being creative. Try it, and, odds are, you'll find that you're better at it now than you were as a kid, says Dr. Adams-Price. As we get older, we get better at expressing ourselves and at judging the interests of our audiences, she says.

Try telling or writing stories about your experiences, she suggests. Recall some significant event in your life and write about it or tell someone about it. (If you're feeling shy, tell your story to a kid.) Tell your story even if you're not sure what it means, Dr. Adams-Price says. In telling and retelling these stories, she notes, we discover new meaning in our lives.

Celebrate your birthday. Children enjoy birthday parties because they know what birthday parties are about. Birthday parties aren't about worrying that you're a year older. They're about having a good time with people you love.

Birthdays are times to celebrate the pleasure of being alive, says Dr. Deitch. So take the opportunity to celebrate. Throw a party. Invite your favorite people. Pop some corks.

Hang out with kids. The best way to experience the world as a magical, wondrous, awe-inspiring place is to spend time with a kid, says Dr. Gottlieb. You don't have to be a parent to do this, of course. You can be a scoutmaster, a Big Brother or Sister, or a volunteer at the local elementary school, he says.

"Spend time with children, and not only will it show you the world through their eyes, I guarantee it will contribute to your sense of purpose," he says.

When you're with kids, remember to pay attention. Listen to them. Ask them questions about their thoughts. Ask about spiritual issues, he suggests. "Children have a kind of spirituality, a kind of awe at the world, a sense of the Godliness of the world, that we have literally forgotten," he says. "It would behoove us to become their students."

Massage: Bodywork for Your Mind and Soul

Massage.

What an evocative word. Second only, perhaps, to hot-fudge sundae. Okay, so that's three words, but you understand. When you think massage, you think strong, sure hands gliding along your body, manipulating muscles, perhaps lingering on a particularly recalcitrant knot or two.

But if you've never experienced a professional massage, the word may also conjure vaguely unsettling images of oils, scents, soft music, and—heaven help us—total nudity.

Let's say you've even been so bold as to look in the phone book or check out the business cards on the bulletin board at your local racquet club or health spa or even hair salon. Unfamiliar terms—from the seemingly straightforward *therapeutic massage* to the threatening *deep muscle* to the downright frightening *craniosacral*—jump out like Dobermans, keeping you warily circling the bodywork boundaries.

The truth is, there are more than 80 recognized types of massage modalities, and even professional therapists don't agree where the lines are drawn among those types. Massage therapy is reputed to help relieve stress, treat muscle injury, reduce swelling, and relieve pain. Since it increases blood flow and relaxation, which decreases blood sugar levels and relaxes the airways, massage therapy may even help chronic problems like diabetes and asthma.

To shed some light on the murky mysteries of massage, *Prevention* writer Michele Morris, on assignment from the magazine, tried out four of the most commonly used (according to the American Massage Therapy Association) massage therapies: Neuromuscular Massage Therapy (NMT), Shiatsu, deep-tissue, and Swedish. If you're thinking of trying it yourself and wondering what to expect, here's a first-person, front-line report on each of these experiences.

Neuromuscular Massage: Spot Therapy

My first session is with Lynn McNutt Cunningham, a former physician's assistant who took up massage about four years ago.

Lynn is dressed in loose batik pants and a simple peach sweater, and she moves with the relaxed sureness of an athlete. While assessing my posture and movement, she tells me that neuromuscular, or trigger-point, massage focuses on spots where muscle fibers, damaged by physical exertion or chronic tension, have adhered to each other or to surrounding tissue or bone. As a result, the fibers no longer extend and contract properly.

By manually breaking up these adhesions and freeing the muscle fibers, says Lynn, the therapist can increase the blood—and consequently, oxygen—reaching the fibers and improve the removal of waste products that cause muscle fatigue and discomfort. Second, judicious pressure on the painful area essentially overloads and short-circuits the nerve impulses. Both actions help eliminate spasms and pain, not only at the site of the adhesion, but often in other areas served by the same nerve pathways—enabling the fibers to work as they were intended.

After Lynn determines that I'm relatively free of postural and structural imbalances, she leaves the room while I take off my clothes. I lie face down on the padded table, hastily arranging the sheet over my nude body. When she returns, Lynn lowers the lights, rubs a little oil on her smooth, warm hands, and then goes to work finding my own private trigger points.

Though the ideal candidate for neuromuscular massage therapy is anyone with specific, chronic pain—Lynn says that she has successfully used it to alleviate symptoms ranging from TMD (temporomandibular disorder) to headaches and "just about any sports injury where there's muscle spasm or swelling"—virtually anyone can benefit from the technique since we all harbor areas of tension and overuse of which we may not even be aware.

For a solid hour, Lynn's hands move surely and gracefully, at one point finding a spot on my neck that I can feel releasing—just like a fist unclenching—deep in my skull, about an inch west of my right ear. The strokes are short and specific, meant to free tissue and enhance blood supply right where it's needed. She lingers on certain spots for a few seconds with gentle but insistent pressure, leaves them for other areas, and revisits them later. Each time, I feel the tissues becoming more pliable and yielding. Some troubled areas—across my upper back and shoulders—I know about; others, down by my hips and the back of my pelvis, are new and surprise me with the immediacy of their soreness.

When I get home and walk around, it's as though my joints have been lubed, with fresh grease injected into the sockets of my hips and shoulders. I smell faintly of coconut and am at once relaxed and energized.

I could get addicted to this.

Shiatsu: Going with the Flow

My second session is with Lisa Baas, a Shiatsu practitioner. I knew I was in for something different when she told me to wear loose-fitting cotton clothing so as not to interfere with the "magnetic, electrical flow around the body."

The one massage modality I tried that didn't require disrobing, Shiatsu is a Japanese form of acupressure—acupuncture without needles—that really falls into a different category than the Western methodologies that most of us associate with massage. There's none of the oil, lotions, or even stroking that people normally associate with massage. Instead, Lisa uses her hands, elbows, knees, and even feet to press various points along 12 energy pathways that are known as meridians, which Shiatsu practitioners believe are instrumental in keeping the "chi," or life force, flowing in proper balance.

Lisa begins by asking my date of birth and posing questions about my activities, stress, recent injuries, eating habits, aches or pains, medications, menstruation—all while examining my posture and hands. While it's not essential that you answer such questions, they are integral to the Eastern approach to the body as a holistic system of energy, flesh, and bone. Lisa then seats me in an ergonomic "kneeling" chair and prods my shoulders and neck on up into the base of my skull. She rotates my arms and tilts my head from side to side, then directs me to lie down on the futon on the floor.

While I lie on one side, then the other, and finally on my back, Lisa manipulates my shoulders, presses up and down along my spine, and at one point slowly pushes her knee into the small of my back while gently pulling my arm backward across my body. She straddles my body and pulls upward on my legs.

I'm sure that it does me some good, but I feel strangely detached during this massage session; more like I'm being worked on than worked with. Call me a parochial Western skeptic, but when Lisa starts talking about sore spots in my back being related to a weakness or lack of energy available to my heart and lungs (which might show up as stress or allergies), she loses me.

Deep-Tissue Massage: The Wailing Trapezius

The music should have tipped me off before my deep-tissue massage with Karol Benson Thomas even started. Kyoko Takazawa's energetic rendition of a French violin concerto filled the tiny massage room in a local tanning salon.

Barefoot and solidly built, wearing a clean white smock and a mass of gray-tinged curly black hair pulled atop her head, Karol asks if the music is okay, then dives right in—kneading, pressing, and stroking. As with the NMT session, this one starts with me on my stomach under a flannel sheet, my face resting in a special cradle at the top of the massage table. The Stradivarius moans; my trapezius wails. "This isn't what I'd call a really deep massage," says Karol, vigorously working my muscles. She adds that it wouldn't be appropriate to apply that kind of pressure after two other massages sandwiched around an active weekend.

"This is about your limit, right?" she says, seemingly trying to reach my sternum by pushing a finger through my back.

I inhale deeply, exhale slowly. "Yes," is all I can manage to say.

Using her elbow and knuckles as well as her fingers to get deep into the muscle, Karol sometimes works against the grain of resistant muscle to loosen any adhesions—a technique similar to NMT that she calls cross-fiber friction. She uses it along my shoulder blades, then up into my neck. And when she finishes, I definitely know that I've been worked over.

Although there's some disagreement about just what deep-tissue massage does, some experts feel that it brings damaged, oxygen-starved muscles the blood they need to heal, while the mechanical action of the stroking and pulling literally helps the body flush out by-products like lactic acid, which is linked to muscle soreness. It also seems to assist in moving lymph—a substance that transports excess fluid, protein, and waste products—into the bloodstream, where it can be filtered through the liver and the kidneys.

The next night, my body is feeling the effects of too much attention. My neck and the outsides of my hips are sore to the touch, and the tops of my shoulders actually seem swollen. I find out later that soreness for a day or two after a thorough deep-tissue massage is to be expected since it has much the same effect on muscles as a hard workout.

Three down, one to go. I think I may make it.

Swedish Massage: The Foundation

Here's a case where familiarity breeds not contempt, but contentment. Judy Umlauf has been untying the knots in my muscles for more than two years, and it's a welcome relief to stretch out on her familiar table.

Judy knows that this time I want a no-frills Swedish massage, but her response echoes that of every other practitioner I've seen: She'll give me what my body needs. After 13 years as a massage therapist, Judy now incorporates several techniques into her practice, though she stuck pretty closely to the basic Swedish strokes at first. "I've been doing this for so long," she says, folding the thick towel to reveal my back, "my hands just know where they need to go and what they need to do."

Judy shifts seamlessly from the gliding effleurage and kneading petrissage strokes of classic Swedish massage to a rhythmic rocking motion called Trager and back again. She even throws in a little "polarity," which, like Shiatsu, is intended to balance the body's energy flow. As I turn onto my back, I realize that Swedish massage is the foundation upon which all the other Western techniques are built. Except for Shiatsu, all of my massages have incorporated variations of these strokes, probably because many massage therapists combine techniques for optimal effect.

After Judy finishes with a light facial massage and her hands hovering slightly above my closed eyes, I'm thoroughly relaxed.

The Message of Massage

So what do I think of massage?

When the final muscle was kneaded and the cap was put on the last bottle of oil, I knew that I was a believer in the value of massage. Even though debates still rage within the medical community about how much massage heals, I don't need a double-blind, doctor-sponsored study to tell me what my hard-working body feels. Every one of these sessions helped me feel more relaxed, more balanced, and sometimes even more energetic than before the laying on of hands.

And that's good enough to make me book my next massage.

Sage Advice

Rx for Staying Sharp

Every time you grab an orange for a snack, buy whole-wheat bread, or take double helpings of carrots, think of it as brain insurance—lifetime brain insurance. Older Spaniards, ages 65 to 90, recently took two tests of mental function. People who got perfect or satisfactory scores turned out to be the ones with the healthiest eating habits. They ate more vegetables and fruit, fiber, vitamin C, folate, beta-carotene, and zinc—and less saturated fat and cholesterol.

Fighting Allergies Can Leave You Beat

When it comes to allergy medicine, "people think that the strong stuff is behind the counter with the pharmacist," says Gary G. Kay, Ph.D., director of the neuropsychology division at Georgetown University Medical Center in Washington, D.C. But Dr. Kay's research shows that in the case of allergy medicines, it's the over-the-counter (OTC) treatments that pack a real wallop. And they can slow us down, he says, without us even realizing it.

Dr. Kay and his colleagues compared people who had or had not each taken a dose of an OTC allergy medicine on tests of attention, memory, and reaction time. Just 90 minutes after the people had taken the recommended doses, "we found enormous differences," he says. Those who had taken the allergy medicine performed much more poorly than the other groups. According to Dr. Kay, the differences were strong enough to be hazardous while driving or to lead to decreased productivity at work. Based on this and other research he has done, Dr. Kay expects to find a similar effect from the antihistamines in nearly all OTC allergy pills.

"You may not notice these differences yourself," Dr. Kay notes. About two-thirds of the people who took the OTC medicine described themselves as feeling fine, but they were just as impaired as those who said the medicine made them feel sleepy.

Dr. Kay recommends that people with allergies who are concerned about this try nonsedating prescription medications. In addition, check with your pharmacist before using any OTC medication with a "P.M." formulation, since it may contain antihistamines to help induce sleep.

Lifting Weights Lifts Your Mood

People with depression actually improved their moods by strength training, according to recent research at Tufts University in Medford, Massachusetts. In fact, the exercise appeared to be as effective as many medications commonly used to treat depression—without the negative side effects. And people even slept better.

These aren't the only perks of weight training. Three different studies have shown that once people become stronger through strength training, they naturally become more physically active. That includes doing more sports and aerobic activities such as dancing, canoeing, golfing, and even gardening. It could be that these activities are easier to do once you are strong. Women also made great transformations in self-confidence—especially when they got stronger than their daughters.

Walk Off Chronic Fatigue Syndrome

Just as a cough can be caused by anything from an allergy to tuberculosis, "a lot of different circumstances can result in what we call chronic fatigue syndrome," explains Quentin Regestein, M.D., who studies chronic fatigue syndrome (CFS) and sleep disorders at Brigham and Women's Hospital in Boston. "Chronic fatigue syndrome is a fruit salad that's flavored by a million different condiments." With so many causes, the illness is particularly difficult to treat.

But a new study offers hope that for some CFS patients, the road to recovery is a walking trail. In a study at St. Bartholomew's and the Royal London Medical School in Britain, researchers enrolled 66 patients in a 12-week program of either aerobic exercise five days a week or flexibility training. By the end of the study, twice as many of the exercisers rated themselves as feeling better compared with those in the flexibility group. The exercising group also showed more improvement on measurements of fatigue.

"It's an optimistic observation," says Dr. Regestein. Since the exercise program consisted mainly of light walking (about 50 percent of maximum heart rate), he suggests that people who want to try this approach "begin with something you know you can do, then build up from there." Dr. Regestein notes that the benefits of exercise for CFS patients may go beyond conditioning the body to fight fatigue. "It is very likely that just getting up and getting out into the daylight regularly helps keep you going."

Being a Workaholic Can Work Out Okay

There may be different types of workaholics, says Marcia Miceli, D.B.A. (doctorate of business administration), professor of human resources at Ohio State University's Fisher College of Business in Columbus. She and two other researchers analyzed more than 50 research articles and books on the topic. Their findings: At least some workaholics are perfectly happy with their status. If you've been putting in long hours beyond what your job actually requires, try asking yourself these questions.

Do my work habits seem excessive—even to me? If you're unhappy with your work habits but can't seem to cut down the extra hours, you may fall into the "compulsive workaholic" category. A licensed therapist can help you work out your problems.

Do I prefer to be in control or to delegate? "We propose that perfectionist workaholics have a strong need to be in control," says Dr. Miceli. Folks with this mindset can do well if they find a job that rewards hands-on management, a high standard of work quality, and the ability to work independently.

Does my job satisfy me? Some people really do seem to find their jobs rewarding even though they spend almost all their time doing them. "These are people who have chosen jobs that enable them to meet their achievement needs and spend a lot of time working at things they really like doing," Dr. Miceli says. Based on clinicians' reports, researchers propose that these achievement-oriented workaholics, if their friends and family are accommodating, may actually experience less stress than their nonworkaholic co-workers.

Maintain-Your-Brain Food

Can one of the omega-3 fats in fish fight Alzheimer's disease? In a study of more than 1,000 people with an average age of 75, those with high blood levels of an omega-3 called docosahexaenoic acid (DHA) were more than 40 percent less likely to develop dementia, including Alzheimer's, over the next nine years than people with low DHA levels. We know that the brain latches onto DHA—its favorite fat—to help build membranes around nerve cells; possibly, the more DHA, the easier it is to zap messages from cell to cell.

At the same time, more omega-3's in your diet may help lift your mood. A study from the University of Antwerp Hospital in Belgium reports that seriously depressed patients had lower omega-3 levels compared with healthy control patients and mildly depressed patients. Why this happens isn't known, but it is known that the brain needs omega-3's to form healthy nerve cells.

Experts advise eating a weekly serving or two of fish rich in omega-3's. A piece of salmon the size of an audiotape will do. Or, for another option, you could try Neuromins, a supplement with 100 milligrams of DHA per capsule. You can take one or two supplements a day. One daily dose supplies about as much DHA in a week as you'd get from one serving of salmon. And, as a bonus for vegetarians, Neuromins is made from tiny sea plants, which is where fish get their omega-3's. It's the first supplement with a nonanimal source of this omega-3. (The other omega-3 in fish is eicosapentaenoic acid, or EPA, which acts as a blood thinner and calms symptoms of inflammatory diseases, such as rheumatoid arthritis. Fish and fish-oil capsules have both DHA and EPA.)

What You Think Affects How You Feel

Nostradamus made a name for himself by forecasting deluges, wars, and other catastrophes. Safe predictions, considering that such things are bound to happen eventually. But when it comes to your health, predicting nothing but the worst can actually make things worse, a new study suggests.

Douglas A. Drossman, M.D., of the University of North Carolina School of Medicine in Chapel Hill, tracked the health of 200 women being treated at a clinic for gastrointestinal problems. Over the course of one year, he found that measurements of health, including pain and number of doctor visits, were considerably poorer in women who exhibited a coping style called catastrophizing. "Catastrophizing describes a profound sense of pessimism and hopelessness," explains Dr. Drossman. A catastrophizer sees herself as a victim of her illness, with no control of the situation. In the study, the catastrophizers had 60 percent more doctors' visits and nearly twice as much pain compared with women with other coping styles.

How do you avert catastrophic thinking? "Keep a positive frame of mind," Dr. Drossman says. "Remind yourself that you're really in control. You can do something about your illness." Simple things like rating your discomfort on a 1-to-10 scale or finding activities to distract you from your illness can put things in perspective and help you feel in control.

Antioxidants May Slow Alzheimer's

They're already being studied for their benefits in cancer and heart disease. Now, a study suggests that two specific antioxidants, vitamin E and a drug called selegiline hydrochloride, may slow the progression of important symptoms of Alzheimer's disease by about seven months.

In a two-year study of 341 people with moderately severe Alzheimer's, two groups given either 10 milligrams of selegiline (Elde-pryl, currently being used to treat Parkinson's disease) or 2,000 international units (IU) of vitamin E daily delayed the loss of the ability to perform daily activities, the progression of severe dementia, and institutionalization.

"We're excited about these results because there are so few options available for people with more severe cases of Alzheimer's," says David Bennett, M.D., associate director of the Rush Alzheimer's Disease Center in Chicago, one of the sites for the study trials. "The benefits of these treatments are small but real—and people can ask for them right now."

Neither selegiline hydrochloride nor vitamin E improved memory or cognitive ability in this study. But two drugs—tacrine hydrochloride (Cognex) and donepezil hydrochloride (Aricept)—are currently being used to treat those symptoms in mild to moderate cases of Alzheimer's.

Note: The doses of vitamin E used in this trial were very high—almost 70 times greater than the current Daily Value of 30 IU. It is essential that doses of this magnitude be monitored by a physician for side effects as well as any progress. A study using low-dose vitamin E supplements showed an increased risk of hemorrhagic stroke.

Back to Sleep

One often-overlooked cause of daytime fatigue is nighttime posture. "Sleeping on your stomach can cause a strain on your back that may be just painful enough to keep you from getting a good night's sleep," says Peter Slabaugh, M.D., spokesperson for the American Academy of Orthopedic Surgeons. For a more restful repose night after night, follow this advice.

- A pillow under your knees comfortably flexes your lower spine, relieving pressure.
- To avoid neck and shoulder aches, use a pillow that's low enough to support your head without flexing your neck. Down pillows work best; foam ones are often too springy.
- Be sure you're warm enough. If you have to stay curled up all night to keep warm, your back is likely to get sore.
- You need enough room to maneuver. "It's normal to move your arms and legs during the night and to roll from side to side," says Dr. Slabaugh. This prevents your joints from staying in one position for too long and getting stiff overnight.
- People who snore or have trouble breathing at night may prefer to sleep on their sides in order to breathe easier.

Can Supplements Keep You Sharp?

Next time you're struggling to decode the directory at the new mega-mall, you might check the whereabouts of the nearest vitamin store. A study at the University of New Mexico in Albuquerque found that healthy supplement users over age 65 scored higher in tests of cognitive abilities, including the types of skills used to read and remember maps like the ones found in malls (skills that doctors call visuospatial skills). Their test results were higher than their nonsupplementing counterparts'.

Smart eating was also connected to performance—participants who maximized their nutrition levels through diet alone performed well, too. But supplementers—even those taking modest doses of multivitamins—appeared to get extra brain boosts. Tests measuring short-term memory and abstract reasoning (the best yardstick of mental pizzazz, according to experts) also suggested a link.

"This study couldn't tell us which nutrients offer this edge, or how they work," says Asenath La Rue, Ph.D., research professor of psychiatry and lead study author, "but it could be that antioxidants somehow slow the normal aging of the brain." This study confirms the oft-seen connection between supplement taking and other good health habits, so other factors could be the fuel behind the brainpower. But it's not a bad idea to regularly top off your healthy breakfast with a multivitamin/mineral tablet and a brisk walk.

Do Missed Workouts Spell Bad Moods?

Aunt Idabell invited herself over to show you how to make borscht, so you can't go for your usual jog through the park. And as you watch her gleefully mashing beets, you realize that you didn't get to work out yesterday either. Or the day before. And you've been crabby all three days. Are you doomed to crankiness every time you miss a workout?

Well, yes, say researchers at the University of Wisconsin–Madison. They tested the mood-altering effects of skipping exercise in 10 volunteers, all of whom were used to working out at least six days a week. The volunteers' moods started to dip by the second no-workout day. Symptoms of anxiety, depression, confusion, and other blahs were common, but the group cheered up again once they went back to working out.

There are many theories as to why exercise has such an impact on mood, says the study's primary author, Gregory W. Mondin, of the department of counseling psychology at the university. They involve everything from body temperature to the psychological effects of changing your routine. The solution is to release the tension, says Mondin. "For some people, the answer may be stretching or even just sitting quietly for a while to relax." Others may feel better after a quick bout of pushups or situps. By the way, this doesn't mean that you're some kind of exercise-a-holic. According to Mondin, "It just means that you're feeling antsy because you didn't work out."

Exercise Right for a Good Night

It's night. Late at night. You've counted so many sheep that the wool is making you itch, but you're wide awake.

Take the time to plan the next day. And write exercise in. In pen. Many studies have found that regular exercise can bring on sound sleep, but they've never focused on people who need sleep most: older adults. A new study found that a four-month program of moderate exercise (four times a week) made for better slumber among a group of sleep-troubled people between the ages of 50 and 76. "There are many factors that keep an older person from sleeping soundly through the night," says Donald Bliwise, Ph.D., of Emory University School of Medicine in Atlanta. One may be changes in body heat. Most people's body temperatures go down at night, but this pattern can become less distinct with age. Exercise may help bring about sleep by causing your body to cool itself down in the hours after working out.

When should you exercise if you want to be out like a light instead of out of your mind? "We generally encourage people to exercise earlier in the day," Dr. Bliwise says. "By rule of thumb, anytime up until dinner-time." Exercising later than that may actually disrupt sleep. He suggests brisk walking, a mild bike ride, or some low-impact aerobics to speed your journey to the land of Nod.

Herbal Elixirs

Boost Your Memory with Ginkgo

Herb expert and Prevention *advisor Varro E. Tyler, Ph.D., Sc.D., describes how this ancient herb may improve memory and (surprise) wake up your sex life.*

If someone you love has Alzheimer's disease, or you want to do everything possible to keep yourself out of its grip, you'll want to know about ginkgo (*Ginkgo biloba*), an ancient herb with a promising future. In China, ginkgo seeds have been used as both food and medicine for thousands of years, but the tree's dried green leaves are the source of the herbal medicine that's making headlines today.

Now a study has confirmed what 20 years of European research has suggested: People who take ginkgo for mild to severe dementia may improve their ability to think and interact with others.

And for people who have cognitive deficiency, a condition caused by inadequate blood flow and nerve damage in the brain, ginkgo biloba extract (GBE) can make a marked improvement in a host of disorienting symptoms such as dizziness, ringing in the ears, headache, memory loss, concentration problems, and confusion.

Here's more good news: Ginkgo can help ease the pain that walking causes for people who have poor circulation in their legs, a condition doctors call intermittent claudication. And there's even mounting evidence to suggest that ginkgo can put back the zing in the sex lives of men whose erections are affected by taking antidepressants.

There are no long-term studies that prove that taking GBE now will prevent Alzheimer's disease or other forms of senile dementia later; such studies would be prohibitively expensive to carry out. But I have neighbors in their sixties who take it regularly and swear by it; they tell me that GBE improves their memories. Since there are no known health risks associated with long-term use of GBE, it's safe to take. The only risk involved is the one to your wallet—good GBE products are relatively expensive.

But don't buy ginkgo as a "smart pill" that improves your intelligence. There's little scientific evidence to show that the herb produces significant benefits for the normal human brain. Sorry about that.

How does ginkgo work? Often with herbs, you can't point to any single compound or mechanism. What we do know is that ginkgo's flavonoids reduce harmful brain effects by preventing the activity of enzymes that produce damaging free radicals (substances that damage cells through oxidation). As antioxidants, flavonoids also scavenge any free radicals that have already been formed.

Finally, terpene derivatives in ginkgo act as bodyguards for the brain, protecting it from blood clots and nerve damage and increasing circulation to the brain.

Unlike synthetic drugs, such as tacrine, commonly prescribed for treatment of dementia, ginkgo is relatively free of side effects. Less than 2 percent of 10,632 people treated with ginkgo reported problems such as mild stomach upsets, headaches, or allergic reactions.

How much should I take? Take 120 to 240 milligrams GBE in two or three separate doses. It works slowly; plan to take GBE for at least eight weeks before you see an improvement. There are no known contraindi-cations to ginkgo, but use it with caution if you're taking anticoagulant herbs (such as garlic, ginger, or feverfew) or a synthetic drug such as warfarin.

What should I buy? Look for ginkgo products with labels that say "24/6," which means the product has been concentrated and contains 24 percent flavone glycosides and 6 percent terpenes.

What should I avoid? Ginkgo is an expensive herb. Standard 40- to 60-milligram tablets typically sell for around $12 for 30 tablets, depending on the brand. Don't buy bargain herbs that sometimes sell for $1 or $2 for the same quantity. There's no guarantee of quality with any herb, but I es-pecially suspect cheap ones.

Avoid using unprocessed ginkgo leaves in any form, including teas; they contain several potent allergens known as ginkgolic acids. These compounds, removed during the processing of GBE, are kissing cousins to urushiol, the chemical that puts the itch in poison ivy.

Ginseng: King of Zing?

Talk about a reputation! Here's an herb that has, at various times throughout history, been believed to boost energy, memory, mood, im-munity, concentration—even conjugation. According to herb expert and *Prevention* advisor Varro E. Tyler, Ph.D., Sc.D., ginseng is considered an adaptogen, a Russian term for products thought to increase a person's resis-tance to stress, fight disease by building vitality, and strengthen normal body functions. (The old-fashioned English word for such an agent is *tonic*.)

That helps explain why you can now find this herb included in everything from gum to snack bars—even coffee. But when it comes to ginseng, it pays to know the real thing. Because, although years of contra-dictory and controversial study results have made it an extremely difficult substance to evaluate fairly, evidence of its ability to recharge the body is now beginning to accumulate.

Based on what we know, Dr. Tyler is convinced that ginseng may have some value as a tonic. And so is Commission E, the German body entrusted with the evaluation of the safety and efficacy of herbal reme-dies. They have decided that ginseng is a "tonic for invigoration and fortification in times of fatigue and debility, for declining capacity for work and concentration, and also during convalescence."

So what do we know? We know a lot about its history, botany, chemistry, and even its effects in small animals. But there is much less sound information on its effects in people. True, there have been clinical trials reporting generally favorable results in terms of health improvement, physical and mental capacities, and various metabolic measurements, with minimal or no side effects. The catch is that few of these studies would be thought acceptable by today's scientific standards.

Fortunately, there have been several reliable studies in the 1990s. Two investigations—one from Sweden involving 390 people, and one from Mexico with 501 people—showed that ginseng, in combination with vitamins and minerals, resulted in an improved quality of life. Other studies reported improvements in memory and other factors associated with psychological well-being and fatigue reduction. In these scientifically exacting studies, the ginseng used was a carefully measured, standardized extract, G-115, which contained 4 percent ginsenosides.

Will the Real Picker-Upper Please Stand Up?

Just because the word *ginseng* appears on a product doesn't mean you're getting the real thing. A host of imitators, hoping to cash in on the reputation of the original, can be found, including Siberian ginseng, Brazilian ginseng, and Indian ginseng. But to be authentic, it must be a species of the genus *Panax*, such as Asian (*Panax ginseng*) and American (*Panax quinquefolius*).

Stick to the genuine article, advises Dr. Tyler, because whatever physiological effects ginseng produces are probably due to a complex mixture of chemicals called ginsenosides found in those. That's why the whole root, or an extract, is so highly valued—and expensive. (Ginseng ranges from about $28 to more than $200 per pound, depending on quality.)

A No-Zap Zing

Studies looking at ginseng's safety have stirred controversies—unnecessarily. For example, in 1979, R. K. Siegel, a researcher at the University of California, Los Angeles, reported toxic side effects, which he dubbed "ginseng abuse syndrome." His findings, based on faulty experimental procedures, have since been discredited. Most other reports of ginseng toxicity have been traced to mislabeled or adulterated products. If you decide to try ginseng, purchase a product that is standardized on the basis of its ginsenoside content. Of the many products on the market, the concentrations of the ginsenosides may vary from about 4 percent to 7 percent. Follow dosage instructions on the label. The recommended dose of a typical product containing 4 percent ginsenosides is two 100-milligram capsules daily.

Ginseng should be combined with a healthy lifestyle that includes exercise, good nutrition, and sufficient sleep. It's not going to cure a lifetime of "don'ts," but it may provide additional benefits to the aforementioned "do's." For beating stress and fighting fatigue, it appears that the herb must be taken continually or it may lose its effectiveness. (If you don't like the idea of always taking pills, try reducing the dosage or stop taking it after a few months and see how you feel.) Another way to use ginseng is to take it during particularly hectic times for an added boost of energy.

Worrywarts and St.-John's-Wort

St.-John's-wort (*Hypericum perforatum*), the herb that is widely used to treat mild depression, has also stirred some controversy. Is it true, as some have claimed, that this herb can cause liver problems?

According to herb expert and *Prevention* advisor Varro E. Tyler, Ph.D., Sc.D., there is no scientific or clinical evidence supporting the assertion that consumption of normal therapeutic amounts of St.-John's-wort causes liver toxicity.

In a study of 3,250 people taking a concentrated extract of the herb three times daily for four weeks, the most common side effects—each reported in fewer than 20 people—were gastrointestinal symptoms, allergic reactions, and fatigue. Notably absent from the list of adverse reactions was any report of liver toxicity.

The rumor about liver problems with St.-John's-wort may stem from the use of large quantities of the herb, along with high doses of other drugs, for its potential anti-HIV activity, says Dr. Tyler. Such cases would certainly not be typical of normal therapeutic use of the herb for its antidepressant effect.

Wary of Valerian?

Another herb that has raised some eyebrows is valerian (*Valeriana officinalis*), a tea that can help you sleep if you drink it before bedtime. Some scientists have questioned its safety—but according to herb expert and *Prevention* advisor Varro E. Tyler, Ph.D., Sc.D., you can "rest easy" if you enjoy a sip of valerian before you tuck in for the night.

The greatest drawback of valerian tea is probably its odor, says Dr. Tyler. There is no scientific evidence that the drink is unsafe. Several years ago, a few scientists expressed concern when certain constituents of valerian known as valepotriates affected the hereditary genes and caused mutations in certain bacteria.

However, valerian tea contains little, if any, valepotriates, which aren't readily absorbed during digestion anyway. In one experiment, only 0.1 percent of the valepotriates originally present in valerian root was found in the tea, and in another study, none could be detected. Commercial preparations (capsules, liquid extracts, and so forth) of valerian usually contain negligible amounts of valepotriates because valepotriates are unstable compounds, decomposing rapidly in storage.

"Therefore, I agree with the German Commission E (the body responsible for evaluating the safety and efficacy of botanical medicines) finding that valerian is a safe and effective sedative and sleep promoter," says Dr. Tyler. "If you find the tea effective, and its unpleasant odor not too bothersome, there is no reason for concern."

part 6

**Break
Free
from Pain**

Making Sense of It All

Backaches, headaches, toothaches. Muscle soreness, joint pain, cramps. All of us hurt at one time or another. What do you do when you're in the throes? If you're like most, you reach for one of those over-the-counter (OTC) pain stoppers. But which one? It was easy when aspirin was the only choice. Today, there are so many different kinds and combinations. How do you choose? On the other hand, where do you go if you're in the market for a natural alternative?

Here's all the latest info you need to make smart decisions.

The good news is that research is uncovering new ways to chase pain without drugs. In fact, it appears that nature's best painkiller may be your own mind—if you know how to use it. In fact, a panel of experts organized by the National Institutes of Health recently declared that deep relaxation may be as effective as drugs and surgery when it comes to relieving chronic pain. Read all about this and learn a pain-relief technique that works for thousands in "Pain Relief without Pills."

Check out the chapter "Is Your Aspirin Making Your Head Hurt?" You may be surprised to learn that taking painkillers for more than two or three days a week on a regular basis could result in a kind of rebound effect. In other words, the pills that you're taking to stop a throb may actually give you a headache. Who would have thought?

Herbal research has uncovered some pretty potent pain-relieving plants. In an exclusive excerpt from his book *The Green Pharmacy*, herb expert, James Duke, Ph.D., offers herbal prescriptions for everything from toothaches to arthritis. If you suffer from migraines, you won't want to miss his report on feverfew, the herb that can actually stop a migraine in its tracks.

Positive Action Plans

Pain Relief without Pills

There should be a mirror up there on the painkiller shelves, right next to all the boxes blaring things like "extra-strength," "buffered," and "timed-release." Because you may already be holding the real key to pain relief—in your mind.

For years, doctors have been prescribing painkilling drugs to people afflicted with chronic backaches, headaches, and joint aches. And, much of the time, the medications worked. Backs unkinked, heads cleared, and joint pain backed off. But stomachs have not been so grateful; erosion of the stomach lining is an all-too-common side effect of painkiller therapy.

So it's big news to think that there's a way to chase chronic pain without drugs. It's even bigger news to know that nature's best pain reliever may be your own mind—if you know how to use it.

A prestigious panel of experts organized by the National Institutes of Health recently declared that deep relaxation may help relieve chronic pain as readily as drugs and surgery do. This marks a major departure from traditional medical thought in the United States. For the first time ever, some of the most renowned medical experts in North America officially recognized that relaxation is a valid treatment—perhaps even the treatment to try first—for lower-back pain, headaches, arthritis, and other chronically painful disorders. And, unlike painkillers and operations, this kind of relaxation requires fewer doctor visits and has fewer side effects: Nobody has ever suffered an eroded stomach lining as a result of sitting down and focusing on his breathing.

Lest you think this declaration comes from some companies trying to sell cassettes of recorded water sounds, understand that relaxation as pain treatment was embraced by truly mainstream doctors reporting in the renowned *Journal of the American Medical Association*.

Just what type of relaxation are they talking about? It's not the kind of relaxation you get from vegging out in front of reruns of *Sisters* with a cup of chamomile tea. It goes deeper than that. In fact, people who med-

(continued on page 188)

Troubleshooting Guide
for the Reluctant Relaxer

Relaxing isn't easy at first, and some folks may be uncomfortable with the idea of deep relaxation or meditation. To make things easier, follow this beginner's guide to total relaxation.

You won't have to twist yourself into a pretzel, subscribe to a new spiritual theory, or do anything far out. This is about relaxation, and it feels good. Promise.

Problem: I just can't seem to relax on command.

Solution: Sure you can; it just takes practice, says Dennis C. Turk, Ph.D., professor of anesthesiology and pain research at the University of Washington School of Medicine in Seattle. "Relaxation is an acquired skill."

Problem: I have trouble with visualization. Me lying on a beach? I can't imagine that, even if Mel Gibson were purring in my ear about the sun caressing my body.

Solution: Put a visualization tape in your stereo or Walkman. "Find the tape that works for you," says Dr. Turk. "What's relaxing and pleasant for me may not be for you. For example, once I made a tape for a guy to help him envision skiing down a mountain on a lovely, cold, sunny day. It was right for him, but to me, a cold, sunny day is when I'd like to be inside by a fireplace."

Problem: I just get frustrated with relaxation audiotapes. They're too new-agey for my taste.

Solution: Another trick that works well is to focus on a scent, a picture, or a candle flame. If you have a heart rate monitor, you might even concentrate on your pulse on the wristwatch that accompanies it. Or, try to sweat away your physical tension with exercise, suggests Margaret A. Caudill, M.D., Ph.D., co-director of the Arnold Pain Center at Beth Israel Deaconess Medical Center in Boston and author of *Managing Pain before It Manages You*. Downshifting through yoga, tai chi, or gentle stretches also helps.

Jon Kabat-Zinn, Ph.D., director of the University of Massachusetts Stress Reduction Clinic in Amherst and one of the forerunners in bringing "mindfulness meditation" into the mainstream, recommends a body scan. "Bring moment-to-moment awareness to each region of your body, starting with your feet, then moving up your legs and torso, then to your hands and arms, and ending with your neck and head. As you encounter areas of discomfort and pain, try intentionally relaxing and softening around them. Try to sense your breath moving in and out through all regions of your body." Whatever method you choose, you should not expect instant results. Cultivating relaxation takes a certain amount of effort and discipline, especially in the early stages of learning.

Problem: I'm in too much pain to think of a pretty scene.

Solution: Try something easier, suggests Dr. Turk, like focusing on your breathing as you think of the letters c-a-l-m in blue neon light. "That's what works for me."

You also might want to change positions, perhaps sitting instead of lying down, or vice versa, Dr. Caudill says.

Problem: Errant thoughts keep encroaching and diverting my attention.

Solution: If your mind still chatters like a teenager on the phone, keep a pad nearby so you can jot down your thoughts. Eventually, you'll run out of ideas and worries, and your mind will clear. Or, try visualizing a basket and imagining that you are stuffing all of your concerns and pain into it and closing the lid, Dr. Caudill says. Whatever you do, don't blame yourself if you can't clear your mind, she adds. "If you judge yourself, you create a feeling of failure. And you don't need that."

Problem: I feel vulnerable when I lie there with my eyes closed.

Solution: Keep your eyes open, leave the lights on, and lock your door. Remember, this isn't as difficult as it may seem. Do what makes you feel relaxed and comfortable.

Keep in mind, relaxation is not about wiping out your thoughts and feelings. It's about making room for calmness and peace in your life.

"People think that deep relaxation is about trying to find a special switch in their mind that shuts things off or puts them in a 'special state.' But everyone's mind goes all over the place," says Dr. Kabat-Zinn. "We tell our patients that we are going to teach them how to be so relaxed that it is okay to be tense at times and to just experience that. Trying to make everything that you don't like go away can be unrealistic and self-defeating."

With deep relaxation comes enhanced calmness. "You'll find a greater sense of self-confidence, knowing you're more in charge of your life and pain," he says. "Deep relaxation isn't a magic pill you take, but a way of being."

itate might recognize some of the relaxation techniques that we're talking about here. But you don't have to attain nirvana to get relief. The total relaxation we're talking about falls somewhere between the couch and the meditation pillow.

It's a simple state of mind to achieve if you know the tricks. First, you break the train of everyday thoughts that induce stress by focusing on the repetition of a word, sound, thought, or breath. Second, you passively disregard other thoughts. Think of them as bumblebees buzzing around your head on a summer day. If you swat, you'll only make the bees angry and persistent. But if you ignore them, they'll buzz a bit and move on.

Like stress, relaxation works from the inside out. As you unwind, your body takes a 180-degree turn, switching from arousal to recuperation. Muscles relax, breathing slows, and your metabolism and blood pressure drop, says Herbert Benson, M.D., president of the Mind/Body Institute and director of behavioral medicine at Beth Israel Deaconess Medical Center, both affiliated with Harvard Medical School, and associate professor of medicine at the medical school.

In contrast, when you're anxious, your body prepares to fight or flee. Your muscles tense, your blood pressure rises, your breathing races, and your pain threshold falls. It doesn't take too many traffic jams and toddler tantrums for your body to be tighter than your clothes after the holidays.

Deep relaxation can short-circuit not only pain but also the emotions that accompany pain, says Dennis C. Turk, Ph.D., professor of anesthesiology and pain research at the University of Washington School of Medicine in Seattle. "The worst thing is to feel helpless, that there's nothing you can do, like when you wake up at 3 A.M. with a terrible headache or back pain. You lie in bed thinking about how miserable you are. If you can use these types of relaxation techniques to gain some sense of control, that, in itself, can reduce some of the stress and discomfort you experience."

Relaxed: How to Get There from Here

"Oh, just relax." That sounds easy, but for many of us, it's not. To succeed, start by lying down or sitting (with your back fairly straight, feet flat on the floor, and hands in your lap) in a darkened room, preferably one that's quiet and without distractions.

Close your eyes and breathe through your nose. Concentrate on your breathing. Make sure you are "belly-breathing"—that is, forcing your belly to expand before your chest rises. This ensures that you are bringing air deep into your lungs. As you breathe out, imagine all tension in your body and mind leaving through your breath.

At this point—just like at night when your head hits the pillow—you'll probably notice your mind darting from every unpaid bill to every gained pound to every unfinished task.

That's where the repetition of a word, such as *one, peace, love,* or *shalom* comes in, says Dr. Benson, the architect of the famed "relaxation response." You can focus on the rhythm of your breath, riding its waves as if you were a raft bobbing on a river. When extraneous thoughts show up, reel them in like fish. Catch them, admire them, then plop them on the bottom of the boat and return to fishing—er—relaxing.

You might find it easier to unwind if you simply reflect on what you are thinking and feeling right now, in the present moment. Audiotapes that help you cultivate this awareness (sometimes by painting a serene scene, such as a mountain, a lake, or a stand of trees) can help beginners, says Jon Kabat-Zinn, Ph.D., director of the University of Massachusetts Stress Reduction Clinic in Amherst and one of the forerunners in bringing "mindfulness meditation" into the mainstream. "Guided meditation tapes are like training wheels—once you learn, you don't need them," he says. "Even so, many of our patients still use the tapes from our clinic 10 to 15 years later."

Classes in relaxation also are available. Check at your local hospital or look under "stress reduction" or "meditation instruction" in the Yellow Pages.

But you can relax just as well at home with a guided-imagery tape, and you won't be subjected to the heavy breathing of a stranger next to you. Whatever your approach, once you've relaxed for 10 to 20 minutes, count to three and slowly open your eyes.

Dr. Benson and other experts suggest an initial goal of one full relaxation session daily. Ideally, build a habit by unwinding each day at the same time. "You might find that if you do it right before bedtime, it's a good way to drift into sleep," says Margaret A. Caudill, M.D., Ph.D., co-director of the Arnold Pain Center at Beth Israel Deaconess Medical Center in Boston and author of *Managing Pain before It Manages You.* "Or, you might find it a good way to start the day—with a clear mind."

Once you've made it routine, you can add impromptu sessions as pain arises, says Jim Spira, Ph.D., licensed psychologist and director of the

Institute for Health Psychology in San Diego. "It's such a simple technique that it can be practiced on airplanes, subways, and in the office. If you wake up in the middle of the night because of pain, you can get into a comfortable chair, practice your technique, and then return to bed."

You'll get even more out of your daily session if you take a break for a few seconds every hour to relax your jaw, breathe deeply, and loosen your tight shoulders, says Dr. Caudill. "By doing this, you won't have 24 hours worth of tension to dissipate at once."

Don't expect more serious types of pain to go away quite so quickly. Studies suggest that you can expect arthritis, back, or other severe pain to lessen after about a month of regular relaxation sessions. It also takes that long for the benefits to start lasting all day, as your body changes its response to stress hormones. Before you realize it, you'll transform from a coiled snake to a lounging cat.

But unlike in an animal, such languor isn't inborn, Dr. Caudill says. "You have to practice constantly in the beginning so you develop a protection against the fight-or-flight response to stress."

Soothe Stabbing Heel Pain: A Three-Part Plan

You swing your feet to the floor—then, ouch! A needlelike pain shoots up your heel. But as you tentatively pad around the house, you notice that the pain is easing. "Thank goodness," you sigh: You've been walking every day for your new weight-loss program and you don't want anything to hinder your progress. Heading out for your sunrise walk, you're reassured when the pain disappears completely. But when you stand up after breakfast just an hour later—ouch! What gives?

In 1998, the *USA Today* annual foot-health hotline received 1,800 calls in one day. The most common complaint? Painful heels. So what is the deal?

The most common cause of stabbing heel pain like this (hurting more after rest, easing with movement) is plantar fasciitis (fash-ee-EYE-tis). The coming-and-going nature of this pain seems downright mysterious—until you know what causes it and how to prevent it.

Fast Aid

Oral anti-inflammatory drugs like aspirin or ibuprofen may help reduce inflammation and curb your heel pain. So can icing the sore area for 10 to 20 minutes. "But this is a 'mechanical' problem," says Glenn Gastwirth, D.P.M., deputy executive director of the American Podiatric Medical Association in Bethesda, Maryland. "If you correct your foot movement, you may not have to do much more. If you have significant inflammation and you seem to be doing everything right, your doctor may consider a steroid injection to offer symptomatic relief. But it's not going to cure the problem and it is not necessarily considered a first course of treatment. Surgery is also something that can be considered, but only when all other treatments fail to help."

The Heel-Calf Connection

The plantar fascia is a sheath of tissue that originates in the base of the heel, continues forward across the sole of the foot, and attaches to the bones in the front of the foot. It stretches and lengthens when you stand on your foot and shortens when your foot is in a relaxed position (when you're sleeping, for example). Plantar fasciitis—that stabbing pain in your heel—strikes when the tissue stretches beyond its normal limits.

The origin of this pain, however, can lie a bit north of your foot: If you exercise without stretching, or if you wear high heels constantly, the muscles of your calf and Achilles tendon (which attaches your calf muscles to your heel) can become tight or shortened. When this happens, your foot must overdo its normal rolling motion in order to make full contact with the ground as you walk. This excessive motion can in turn overstretch and irritate the plantar fascia.

Overstretching Tears Tissue

Every time you take a step, your foot flattens out. "The rolling of the foot inward over the arch, called pronating, is a natural movement that makes the foot elongate," explains Glenn Gastwirth, D.P.M., deputy executive director of the American Podiatric Medical Association in Bethesda, Maryland. "It's excessive pronation that causes problems."

Tiptoe Off

Curious fact: If you walk on tiptoe, you may feel temporary relief from plantar fasciitis. That's not because your heel is off the ground, but because you are shortening the plantar fascia again and therefore easing the pressure on it. That's why women who regularly wear high heels can feel relief from heel pain when wearing them. And it's another good reason to stretch your calves regularly.

When the Achilles tendon or calf muscles are tight, the soft tissue of the plantar fascia stretches too far. It gets tiny tears, which become irritated and inflamed. You go to sleep, and the tissue retracts as the foot relaxes to its natural position. Then when you put your weight on it as you step out of bed, the fascia gets a sharp or sudden tug as your arch flattens, reirritating the injured tissues.

One thing that can help is if you remember not to tuck yourself in at night until you've placed some shoes by your bed. "The foot does its best healing overnight, while it's not bearing any weight," says Kurt Jepson, a physical therapist in Saco, Maine. "Standing up on an unsupported foot during the middle of the night or first thing in the morning can stress the injured area and wipe out any healing that has taken place."

To minimize that risk, slip your feet into supportive shoes before they hit unforgiving ground. Make sure that the shoes have sturdy arch support and are always in plain view. The best shoes won't do anybody any good if they're kicked under the bed.

A little walking will gradually stretch that tissue, so the pain subsides. That, of course, may make you feel good enough for a "real" walk. But unless you get to the root of the problem, that will only reinforce the cycle of injury. Luckily, you can prevent this pain chain reaction as simply as one, two, three.

#1: Stretch, Stretch, Stretch

It's the number one defense against heel pain caused by plantar fasciitis. Stretch your calves slowly and smoothly (don't bounce or jerk) every day after you warm up and after your walk. If you're in pain now, stretch at least three times a day, before and after you walk.

Stick with it. "When people tell me that they're stretching and they still have pain," says Dr. Gastwirth, "often it's because they're really not stretching as reliably as they say." Do it religiously.

#2: Use the Right Shoes

Besides keeping your feet safe from all the nasty stuff down there, good walking shoes keep your feet stable and prevent excessive pronation. Here's how to get the best pain protection.

Buy new shoes regularly. If you have heel pain, replace your walking shoes after 300 to 350 miles—a little sooner than the 500 miles recommended for people without foot problems. Although they may still look good, they're not providing the same cushioning and support that they did when new. Here's Dr. Gastwirth's suggestion: Buy a new pair every 150 miles. (For example: If you walk 10 miles a week, mark your calendar to buy another new pair of shoes in 15 weeks.) At that point, begin to alternate the new pair with your current pair. That way you'll always be supported by shoes that are in great shape. In another 150 miles, discard the older pair and buy a new one.

Choose good-fitting walking shoes with firm heel counters. Heel counters are the back parts of the shoes (not the sole), which surround your heel. If they're fairly stiff and supportive, they can help control foot motion and excessive pronation. A good fit is one that's not too tight, yet does not allow any slipping up and down as you walk.

Check your shoes often for abnormal wear and tear. Put your shoe on the table: If you see that the heel counter is mashed down on one side, the sole is worn at an angle, or any pattern of excessive wear, it's time for a new pair—now.

Get good arch support. You may want to add arch supports to your other shoes if you're in pain. Supporting your arch also helps keep your foot from rolling in. Over-the-counter (OTC) arch supports may be just as effective as prescription orthotics in some cases. Give the OTC ones a try first.

Check out other foot aids. Heel pads, cushioned insoles, and heel cups—available at most pharmacies—can help provide temporary relief from pain. Heel cups can add some support and cushioning to a less supportive shoe as well as compensate for thinning fat pads in the foot that come with aging. But keep in mind that you won't find a permanent

Heavy Heels?

An irony for anyone walking for weight loss is that excess pounds may themselves be a factor in heel pain. It's also why getting the very best shoes and stretching every day is extremely important. See a professional shoe fitter when you shop. (If you fail to see improvement after several weeks on this sort of program, consult an orthopedist or podiatrist.)

solution on the drugstore shelf. For longer-lasting relief, what you really need is to control foot motion.

#3: Watch Your Workouts

If you have heel pain, cut back on your weekly mileage. Remember, although a walk may ease pain as your foot stretches out, real healing takes time. You may not have to stop completely, but you should adjust your walking, to avoid the following:

Hiking. The uneven terrain will push your foot off center and may aggravate your condition.

Uphill walking. Tackling hills may put more stress on the inflamed tissue. Downhill is okay, but if you'd have to come back up, find a new route.

Sloped striding. If you've been walking on the side of a sloped road, you may have forced one foot to excessively pronate. Find a sidewalk route so you can walk on a flat surface.

Too much, too soon. Not that you'll never be able to walk long distances again, but if you gear up too fast, you won't have time to notice the problem until the pain is full-blown again. Increase mileage or speed very gradually.

Is Your Aspirin Making Your Head Hurt?

Headaches are Joan's weakness. She gets them. She's read about them. She knows the ugly muggers inside and out. Or thought she did.

Joan had occasional migraines for years. But about five years ago, they seemed to become more frequent—two, three, four times a month. She auditioned every remedy that came down the pike, but couldn't seem to find a drug, prescription or otherwise, to fight them. Eventually, she found one—Imitrex (sumatriptan succinate)—that seemed to work.

"It gave me my life back," she recalls. "But I continued to toss down aspirin at those small twinges—the little migrainey flickers that I didn't want to pop a real pill for.

"So I kept going, twinge followed by aspirin, followed by twinge, followed by aspirin. One day, I heard Harvard neurologist Nathaniel Katz, M.D., on TV explaining that the over-the-counter (OTC) pills you take to get rid of headaches can actually make headaches worse if you take them too often. Then it hit me: 'Hey! You're talking about me.'"

Joan isn't alone. A lot of people with headaches have these sneaky ones that are caused by the very painkillers taken to cure them. "At least 2 percent to 3 percent of the population in this country—millions of people—may use large quantities of pain medications for headache control," says Ninan T. Mathew, M.D., director of the Houston Headache Clinic.

"Whether you call them analgesia-overuse headaches or the more common term, rebound headaches, they're a major health issue that people don't know about," says Dr. Katz, director of chronic pain services at Brigham and Women's Hospital in Boston.

Indeed, Joan didn't know about them. But they can be identified, caught, and treated—if you know that they exist.

Rebound Warning Signs

Here's what should tip you off—and what can alert you that you're head to head with the warning signs of rebound headache.

• You're taking painkillers for migraine or tension headaches more than two or three days a week on a regular basis. This is the limit that most headache experts set for safety of either prescription or OTC headache medicines. (Joan was taking three aspirin at least three times a day, almost every day.) "If you take analgesics more than a couple of times a week for migraine or related headaches, you're vulnerable to having the headaches escalate in frequency and become more difficult to treat," says rebound headache expert Joel R. Saper, M.D., director of the Michigan Head Pain and Neurological Institute in Ann Arbor.

Bonked by the Rebound?

Common over-the-counter (OTC) drugs can trigger rebound headache. Here are some of the most notorious double agents.

Combination analgesics: Painkillers containing caffeine are prime causes of rebound headache because caffeine withdrawal itself triggers headache.

"The good side of caffeine is that it improves the effectiveness of aspirin or Tylenol by about 30 percent, so you need 30 percent less of those medications," says Glen Solomon, M.D., former head of and current consultant to the headache section at the Cleveland Clinic. "But if you overuse painkillers like Excedrin, Anacin, Vanquish, or other caffeine-containing analgesics for migraines, your blood vessels will be chronically constricted from the caffeine. Then, when you stop the caffeine, the blood vessels will dilate and give you a severe headache." Caffeine also is believed to work via brain chemical stimulation. Both mechanisms may contribute to the rebound effect.

Some experts, such as Dr. Solomon, think that only painkillers with caffeine can cause rebound headaches.

Others, like Joel R. Saper, M.D., rebound headache expert and director of the Michigan Head Pain and Neurological Institute in Ann

• You can't leave the house without a bottle of painkillers in your purse or briefcase. (Joan had a stash of aspirin in her purse, in the office, and both upstairs and downstairs at home.)

• You're buying aspirin or acetaminophen as often as you buy *TV Guide* or *Newsweek*.

• When you sleep late on weekends, you wake up with a pounding headache—your body demanding its fix. (Joan avoided sleeping in, because she knew it would give her a headache. But she often woke up with headaches anyway.)

• You have a headache almost daily or get one at the slightest mentally or physically stressful situation.

• Pills don't get rid of the pain, but "they take the edge off." "That phrase—'take the edge off'—should set off a light bulb that what you're dealing with is withdrawal and rebound," says Glen Solomon, M.D., for-

Arbor, feel that "all OTC painkillers are potentially capable of causing rebound."

Aspirin and acetaminophen (like Tylenol): These single-ingredient analgesics are less likely to cause serious rebound than caffeine-containing compounds, and the low-dose aspirin that you take to prevent heart disease won't rebound at all. If you're not headache-prone, you'll probably never develop rebounds from taking these medications.

Non-aspirin OTC nonsteroidal anti-inflammatory drugs (NSAIDs): These are Advil and other forms of ibuprofen, ketoprofen (Orudis KT, Actron), and naproxen (Aleve). They are the least likely to cause rebound headache. In fact, "some data are starting to tell us that they don't seem to induce rebound," says Fred Sheftell, M.D., director of the New England Center for Headache in Stamford, Connecticut, and co-author of *Headache Relief for Women*. But until there are more data, it makes sense to limit these, too. Follow label guidelines. Too much can cause other side effects, such as upset stomach.

Remember, too, that prescription analgesics including Fiorinal (butalbital, aspirin, and caffeine) and Fioricet (butalbital, acetaminophen, and caffeine) can also cause rebound headaches. If you're experiencing any of the rebound warning signs, discuss them with your physician.

mer director of and current consultant to the headache section at the Cleveland Clinic. "It's the universal rebound statement."

Where Is the Logic?

Joan recognized that she was suffering from rebound headache, but she was confused: How could such classic, safe medications as aspirin and acetaminophen cause what they are designed to cure?

One reason may be that OTC analgesic labels tell you how many you can take in a 24-hour period but don't set a limit on how many days a week the medication should be taken. Pain experts say that rebound can occur when you stop taking the painkillers for any period of time (even as short as overnight). Your body withdraws from them, and you get a pounding headache. Its analogous to a regular coffee-drinker who gets a withdrawal headache when she sleeps in on the weekend and misses her two-cup fix.

It's a biological reaction, explains Fred Sheftell, M.D., director of the New England Center for Headache in Stamford, Connecticut, and co-author of *Headache Relief for Women*. Your body gets accustomed to painkillers; then, when they wear off, the enemy returns.

So far, researchers don't yet know exactly how rebounds happen. "There's some indication that frequent headaches alter the brain's chemistry in such a way that it can't handle pain well; it loses the ability to modify pain," says Dr. Mathew. "Chronic use of pain medications further complicates that process and makes the brain more unable to handle pain. Frequent pain medication alters the natural history of headache."

How to Fight a Rebounder

Of course, the first step in fighting these headaches is recognizing that you have them. And since the typical arsenal of headache remedies may be triggering your pain, you need to try these alternative strategies.

Start a diary. A headache diary, that is. Record the time of day that you get your headache and what type of medicine you take to remedy it. "This helps you keep track of what's going on," says Paul Duckro, Ph.D., director of the chronic headache program at St. Louis Behavioral Medicine Institute and co-author of *Taking Control of Your Headaches*. "It's taking pills mindlessly that gets you in trouble. You wonder, 'Oh, did I take one already?' With a diary, you realize how many you're taking."

Charting your painkiller usage will tell you if you're in that semi-weekly (or more) problem zone. And a pill diary helps you pay attention: Overuse won't skulk silently into the medicine cabinet, as it so easily does to the headache-prone.

Quit cold turkey. The only way for the pain machine in your brain to reset itself is to stop feeding it pills. Complete resetting can take anywhere from 4 to 12 weeks, says Dr. Sheftell. That usually means about 7 to 10 days of increased headaches. They're no bag of butterscotch—but they don't bother some folks too much.

Luckily, Joan was one of them. She stopped gulping aspirin once she realized it was messing with her head. She didn't feel bad at all. Not every flicker turned into a migraine. Most of the time, they went away. Now, they're not nearly as frequent.

If you don't fare as well, "the important thing to remember is, if you can just manage to stay off daily pain medicine, you'll feel much better after two to three weeks," says Dr. Mathew.

If Quitting Isn't Going Well

To mollify discomfort, try these headache-management techniques. *Manage* is the magic word. "Headaches are managed rather than cured," says Dr. Duckro.

Take a shower. For some people, a hot shower can sometimes loosen a tension headache and make it go away. Dr. Solomon says that other people find that a cold compress to the forehead or heat applied to the neck makes them feel better.

Rub it away. Massaging the muscles in your shoulders, neck, face, and scalp may relieve headache. If you can get someone to do it for you, great. But when there's nobody available, you can use your own hands, too.

Yoga, meditation, guided imagery (via audiotapes), warm baths, and biofeedback are some more headache tools that may work for you by relieving stress. If they're not enough to see you through withdrawal, a headache specialist or clinic may be able to help you cope.

Sage Advice

Tickle the Keyboard

Anyone who spends long hours at a computer keyboard is at risk for carpal tunnel syndrome, tendinitis, and other work-related upper-extremity disorders. To lower your risk, lighten up.

When researchers used special equipment to measure how hard a group of office workers hit the keys when they typed on computers, they noticed two things. First, everyone used much more force than necessary:

four to five times more, on average, than was needed for the keystrokes to register. Second, those who used the most force had the strongest symptoms of work-related upper-extremity disorders.

It is possible to learn to tap the keyboard instead of pounding it, says study author Michael Feuerstein, Ph.D., professor at the Uniformed Services University of the Health Sciences in Bethesda, Maryland, and Georgetown University Medical Center in Washington, D.C. Here are his suggestions.

• Practice typing with a light touch. Post reminders where you can see them as you work.

• Identify your "triggers." You may tend to type harder when you're tired, hurried, or under stress, for example. Pay extra attention to your keyboard force at those times.

• Check your posture. Keep your wrists relaxed but not bent upward or downward. Be sure that your monitor is at eye level. Correct any problems that put you in an awkward posture.

• Cut back on caffeine. "It's just speculation," says Dr. Feuerstein, "but drinking too many caffeinated beverages could translate to increased tension that might relate to increased force when using the keyboard."

• Listen to your body. Pain, aching, stiffness, burning, tingling, or numbing in your hands, wrists, arms, or shoulders are "signals that something may not be right," says Dr. Feuerstein. See your doctor or an occupational physician, and you may avoid more serious injury later.

Natural Relief for Migraines

If you get migraines, get a whiff of this finding by Alan Hirsch, M.D., director of the Smell and Taste Treatment and Research Foundation in Chicago. In his study of 50 migraine patients, he found that the scent of green apples made headache pain fade.

Migraine pain was found to improve more during an attack when the subjects sniffed tubes containing a green apple smell than when sniffing unscented tubes.

"It could be a distraction effect, so that the subjects were thinking about the smell instead of their pain. Or it could be that the smell actually reduces muscle contractions in the head and neck, reducing the pain," explains Dr. Hirsch.

Why green apples? Previously, Dr. Hirsch found that the smell reduced anxiety. "Since people with migraines say that their headaches worsen when they're anxious, we thought the odor might be helpful." Other pleasant smells might bring relief equally well, and the effect may work on other forms of pain also, he says.

Fight Back Pain

About 15 years ago, a young man learned a martial arts style called chung moo doe. After a few months of practice, his severe back pain, which doctors told him could be eased only through surgery, began to disappear. And it hasn't returned since.

That might be the end of the story, except that the young man became a doctor himself—and created a therapy program for back pain based on the same techniques that helped him. It's called Alt-Med Research Group, and founder Patrick Massey, M.D., Ph.D., says that his treatment center has been phenomenally successful since it opened four years ago at Alexian Brother's Medical Center in Elk Grove Village, Illinois. "Ninety-three percent of people who walk in the doors of our clinic walk out pain-free," he says.

No breaking bricks or chopping boards in half here. Dr. Massey's patients learn flowing, comfortable motions that are performed for about 20 minutes a day. "The body's own movement stimulates circulation and flexibility, accelerating its own healing process," he explains.

A study of 43 sciatica patients, all of whom failed to get relief from standard therapies, found that 91 percent were pain-free after three months in the program. Whether that's the result of increased blood flow to the beleaguered back, increased muscle strength that comes with exercise, or some other reason, the results are impressive.

For now, people interested in the Alt-Med program need to travel to the Chicago area. But Dr. Massey and his team are planning a clinic in Boston in the near future, as well as national seminars. To find out more, contact Alt-Med Research Group, 850 Beisterfield Road, Suite 4011, Elk Grove, IL 60007.

On Your Knees: Try This Instead of Surgery

If you think your knee pain now means knee replacement later, here's some news for you: If you have osteoarthritis, you may be able to skirt the scalpel with a spin on the exercise bike or a walk in the park.

In one study, aerobic exercise (30 to 45 minutes, three times a week) reduced pain and disability levels enough so that people who had osteoarthritis and were considering knee replacement surgery "might be able to put it off for several years," says study leader Walter Ettinger, M.D., professor of internal medicine and public health science at Bowman Gray School of Medicine in Winston-Salem, North Carolina. In some cases, exercise might be able to eliminate the need for surgery altogether.

Of the 439 people with osteoarthritis in the study, aerobicizers reported a 12 percent reduction in knee pain as well as increased mobility when walking, climbing up and down stairs, and getting in and out of cars. Those who lifted weights also reported significant pain reduction and mobility gains.

Exercise may unkink an arthritic joint because it strengthens muscles surrounding the knee, stabilizes the joint, and makes it less susceptible to pain. It may also increase production of pain-blocking endorphins. Finally, as exercisers noticed improvement, they developed an "I can do it" attitude that lessened their perceptions of pain. One note to the newly active: Expect to feel some soreness and pain as your body gets used to being active. But when you stick with it, you'll have less pain over time.

Herbal Elixirs

Nature's Best Pain Relievers

In an excerpt from his book The Green Pharmacy, *herb expert James A. Duke, Ph.D., discusses the best plant-based medicines for pain management.*

The worst pain that I ever had was caused by a slipped disk. It was just like the pain that I'd experienced from time to time with gout—unbearable. My doctor did what doctors do: He gave me potentially addictive pain pills and nonsteroidal anti-inflammatory drugs. I took more drugs for that slipped disk than I had ever taken in my life. I also took more herbs than I'd ever previously taken, trying to minimize the side effects of the pharmaceuticals.

Doctors recognize two kinds of pain, acute and chronic. Acute pain comes on suddenly, typically subsides with time, and usually is alleviated with common pain relievers. Examples would be a headache or the pain of an injury. Chronic pain may begin as acute pain, but it lasts much longer—months or even years—and often cannot be relieved using standard therapies. Those with chronic pain often wind up in a personal hell. Their pain can make them depressed, and with depression, the pain may become worse and more difficult to treat.

If you have persistent pain, see a doctor for a diagnosis. Once the cause has been figured out, rational treatment becomes possible. But if, like many people who have chronic pain, you don't get a clear diagnosis and your pain goes on and on, I'd suggest consulting a pain clinic. These medical clinics, which are relative newcomers to the health care scene, use a variety of drugs and alternative approaches to help you control your pain even if you can't completely eliminate it. Among the alternative approaches used in some pain clinics are exercise, meditation, and biofeedback.

Green Pharmacy for Pain

There are also a number of herbs that can help.

*Clove (***Syzygium aromaticum***).* Dentists around the country recommend clove oil as first-aid for toothache, and in fact, it's what my mother used to give me for toothache. It works, and its use is endorsed by Commission E, the group that advises the German government on herbal medicine. You apply this oil directly to the painful tooth.

*Red pepper (***Capsicum, *various species*).* Red pepper contains pain-relieving salicylates, chemicals that are similar to salicin, the herbal equivalent of aspirin. In fact, red pepper once ranked as the best food-grade source of salicylates, although a new study has downgraded it considerably. This herb also contains capsaicin, a compound that stimulates the release of the body's natural painkillers, called endorphins.

Some folks like the spicy taste of red pepper. I know I do. I suggest using more of this wonderful spice in your cooking.

Capsaicin also works when used externally, by interfering with substance P, a pain transmitter in the skin. So many studies have shown benefits from applying capsaicin externally that the Food and Drug Administration approved pain-relieving skin creams containing 0.025 percent capsaicin (Zostrix, Capzasin-P) for the treatment of arthritis and rheumatism. (If you use a capsaicin cream, be sure to wash your hands thoroughly afterward: You don't want to get it in your eyes. Also, since some people are quite sensitive to this compound, you should test it on a small area of skin to make sure that it's okay for you to use before using it on a larger area. If it seems to irritate your skin, discontinue use.)

Willow (**Salix, various species**). Willow bark contains salicin. In fact, most plants contain some salicin or related salicylates. Just 100 years ago, aspirin was derived from several plants that contain more of these compounds than most: willow, meadowsweet, and wintergreen. When medicines have been in short supply during wartime, doctors in some countries have successfully gone back to using willow bark for pain relief.

Commission E recognizes willow bark as an effective pain reliever for everything from headache to arthritis.

For many kinds of pain relief, I'd start with about a half-teaspoon of salicin-rich willow bark or up to as much as five teaspoons of white willow (*S. alba*), which has a lower salicin concentration. Of course, not everyone knows which species they have, and salicin content varies from species to species. So I'd suggest starting with a low-dose tea and working your way up to a dose that provides effective pain relief.

If you're allergic to aspirin, you probably shouldn't take aspirin-like herbs, either. Also, you should not give either aspirin or its natural herbal alternatives to children who have pain with viral infections such as colds or flu. There's a chance that they might develop Reye's syndrome, a potentially fatal condition that damages the liver and brain.

Evening primrose (**Oenothera biennis**). This herb is one of our best sources of the amino acid tryptophan. In studies, tryptophan supplements have reduced pain caused by acute and chronic illness and also increased people's abilities to tolerate pain. Naturopaths often recommend taking one gram of evening primrose oil four times a day to relieve the pain and nerve damage of diabetic neuropathy, a particularly painful condition that sometimes develops in people with diabetes. I'd suggest taking powdered seeds instead, because evening primrose loses much of its tryptophan in the oil-extraction process.

Ginger **(Zingiber officinale).** Few people think of ginger as a pain reliever, but it is. In one study, researchers recruited 56 people—28 with rheumatoid arthritis, 18 with osteoarthritis, and 10 with the painful muscle condition fibromyalgia—and gave them two to four teaspoons of powdered ginger a day. After three months, more than 75 percent reported significant pain relief with no side effects.

You can also use ginger externally. Hot ginger compresses seem to help relieve abdominal cramps, headache, and joint stiffness. I'd suggest adding hot pepper to these compresses.

Kava kava **(Piper methysticum).** This tropical herb contains two pain-relieving chemicals, dihydrokavain and dihydromethysticin, that have analgesic effectiveness comparable to that of aspirin. Although kava kava has been described as a narcotic, it is nonaddictive. When you chew the leaf, your mouth goes numb. As a result, this plant might be used to relieve the painful symptoms of sore throat, sore gums, canker sores, or even toothache.

Lavender **(Lavandula,** *various species).* Lavender oil is aromatherapy's top treatment for pain, and in fact, this oil was in on the ground floor of aromatherapy's beginnings. In the 1920s, aromatherapy's founder, French perfume chemist Rene-Maurice Gattefosse, happened to burn his hand in a laboratory accident. Plunging his hand into the nearest cool liquid, lavender oil, Gattefosse experienced rapid relief. Since then, researchers have discovered that some essential oils reduce the flow of nerve impulses, including those that transmit pain. In lavender oil, the key constituents appear to be linalool and linalyl aldehyde.

You can mix a few drops of lavender oil in a tablespoon of vegetable oil and massage it into the painful area.

Mountain mint **(Pycnanthemum muticum).** This herb is high in pulegone, a chemical similar to capsaicin that also has pain-relieving effects. I suggest making a tasty tea, then using the spent leaves (or fresh ones) as a poultice on painful areas. Just wait until the leaves are cool—but still wet—and hold them to the area that hurts. (Don't use this treatment if you are pregnant, however.)

Peppermint **(Mentha piperita).** Menthol, the active constituent in peppermint, has anesthetic effects. In one study, scientists asked 32 people who had headaches to massage tincture of peppermint oil on their tem-

Analgetea

Here's a pain-relieving herbal blend to keep on hand: willow bark, red pepper, cloves, ginger, peppermint, and mountain mint. Just mix whichever of these herbs are available in proportions that appeal to your taste. You can use this mixture to make a tea whenever you feel the need, or you can make a poultice to apply directly to painful areas.

ples. This had significant pain-relieving effects. But if you try peppermint oil, be sure to dilute it by adding a few drops to a couple of tablespoons of any vegetable oil. Pure peppermint oil can be irritating to the skin. And never ingest the oil; a very small amount can be toxic.

Sunflower **(Helianthus annuus).** Sunflower seeds are among the best sources of phenylalanine, a chemical involved in pain control. Studies suggest that phenylalanine helps reduce pain by inhibiting the breakdown of enkephalins, chemicals involved in pain perception. In studies with both humans and animals, phenylalanine makes acupuncture more effective at reducing pain. In laboratory rats, the chemical enhanced the effect of morphine and made it last longer.

If I was in pain, I'd eat a handful of sunflower seeds—I'm a habitual seed muncher anyhow—and use ground seeds in a poultice on painful areas.

Turmeric **(Curcuma longa).** Many studies agree that the curcumin in turmeric has anti-inflammatory effects, including a significant effect in relieving rheumatoid arthritis. But it takes more than a shake of the spice jar to gain this benefit. The dose that naturopaths recommend is 400 milligrams three times a day. To get that much, you'd have to consume at least one-third of an ounce of this herb. So if you'd like to try turmeric for pain, I'd suggest taking capsules, even if you have to make your own. (Empty gelatin capsules can be purchased at health food stores.)

Eucalyptus **(Eucalyptus globulus).** Aromatherapists often suggest adding eucalyptus oil to the pain-relieving essential oils of lavender and peppermint. The compound cineole, which is found in eucalyptus, speeds absorption of the other aromatic pain relievers through the skin. Remember, though, that these oils are best reserved for external use only.

Rosemary **(Rosmarinus officinalis).** Commission E recommends using two to three teaspoons of dried rosemary to make a cup of pain-relieving tea. For a bath that will relax you and that may provide pain relief, fill a cloth bag with two ounces of rosemary and toss it into your bathwater.

*Feverfew (*Tanacetum parthenium*).* It's been more than 10 years now since feverfew helped my sister-in-law beat her migraines. This herb also helped my secretary's sister. I consider feverfew one of the most interesting herbs in modern herbalism.

In my own experience, and this is reflected in the medical literature, feverfew works for about two-thirds of those who use it consistently. My sister-in-law's experience is typical. Before she tried feverfew, she averaged about one migraine a week and spent about $200 a year trying to counteract the pain.

Studies published in the *British Medical Journal* agree that taking feverfew regularly prevents migraine attacks. And according to the *Harvard Medical School Health Letter*, "eating feverfew leaves has become a popular method for preventing migraine attacks in England. Some people for whom conventional treatments for migraine have not worked have turned to feverfew with good results." It's nice to know that I'm in such good company on this one.

People who use feverfew often use fresh leaves, typically ingesting one to four leaves a day to prevent migraines. If you have access to the fresh herb, you might try this approach, but don't expect the leaves to taste good. And some 10 to 18 percent of the people who use fresh feverfew develop mouth sores or inflammation of the mouth and tongue.

The good news is that you don't have to eat the leaves to get the full benefits of this herb. You may be able to avoid the side effects by making a tea with two to eight fresh leaves. Steep them in boiling water, but do not boil them. Boiling may break down the parthenolides, ingredients that are thought to stop serotonin from flooding into the brain, forcing blood vessels to open wide and give you a headache.

You can also take this herb in capsules, which is really the easiest way to do it. Depending on the potency of the herb, doses may vary from one capsule a day (60 milligrams) to six capsules a day (about 380 milligrams) of fresh, powdered leaf or two daily 25-milligram capsules of freeze-dried leaf. Feverfew capsules are sold at many herb shops and health food stores. By all means, discuss the herb with your doctor if you have a hard time arriving at an appropriate dose.

One caveat: Pregnant women should not take feverfew, because of a remote possibility that it might trigger miscarriage. And women who are nursing should not use it, because of the possibility of passing the herb to infants in breast milk. Finally, long-term users often report a mild tranquilizing or sedative effect, which may be welcome or unwelcome, depending on your temperament.

Home Remedies

Soothe Tooth Pain with Fluoride

"I used to have sensitive teeth, and eating cold foods caused me more pain than pleasure. Then my mother-in-law suggested that I glaze my teeth with fluoridated toothpaste a few times a day. It worked, and it's great to be able to eat frozen yogurt again!"

Tooth sensitivity occurs when a tooth's enamel gets worn away, exposing a sensitive network of fluid-filled tunnels that lead to the nerve of your tooth. The causes include vigorous brushing and tooth grinding, and acidic foods and drinks.

Toughening up tooth surfaces by dabbing them with fluoride is effective, which is one reason why your dentist does it during a checkup. "At home, rub a heavily fluoridated toothpaste approved by the American Dental Association (ADA) into the sensitive areas of your teeth several times a day," says Geraldine Morrow, D.M.D., past president of the ADA. Look for toothpastes containing 0.15 percent fluoride ion—the maximum amount of fluoride you can get. You may also want to try brushing with a toothpaste made for sensitive teeth. Brands such as Sensodyne contain one of two protective ingredients—strontium chloride or potassium nitrate—that over time will block the painful sensations being sent to your tooth's nerves. Finally, stay away from toothpastes promising to whiten and brighten teeth to a sparkling sheen. Some of those are so abrasive that they can actually erode the enamel on your teeth. And if you have receding gums, which can expose areas of your teeth under the enamel, stay away from tartar control toothpastes as well, says Dr. Morrow. These can also increase the sensitivity of your teeth.

Parsley Ice Cubes for Bruises

"My skin tends to bruise easily, and my favorite sport is racquetball—not an ideal combination, since you're bound to get hit by a ball now and then. After playing a few games, I survey the damage and apply parsley ice cubes to the bruised areas. Thankfully, I can keep playing without looking like a casualty of war."

Parsley has a traditional reputation for dispelling black-and-blue marks, and ice can prevent swelling. Combine the two, and you'll have a bruise remedy at the ready in your freezer, says herbalist Sharleen Andrews-Miller, faculty member at the National College of Naturopathic Medicine in Portland, Oregon, and associate medicinary director at the college's public clinic.

"Just whirl a handful of parsley and about a quarter-cup of water in a blender or food processor until it looks like slush. Then fill ice cube trays half full," she suggests. "Wrap frozen cubes in gauze or thin cloth and apply to bruised spots as needed." Parsley ice cubes also work well for cooling minor burns.

Treat Windburn with TLC

"I walk three miles every day at lunch. But sometimes, the cold wind can be overpowering and make my face feel like a frozen glacier. On days like these, I softly rinse my face with warm water and apply petroleum jelly over particularly sensitive areas. That way I can return to work and not have to worry about my face cracking when I smile."

You don't have to be a skiing or sailing enthusiast to suffer windburn. "Whenever your skin is exposed to severe wind, it loses moisture quickly and becomes dry and chafed, especially if it's cold," says Patricia Farris Walters, M.D., clinical assistant professor of dermatology at Tulane University School of Medicine in New Orleans. "The physical friction of the wind also agitates dry skin."

Snuggling up to a warm compress can provide instant relief. "First, try to gently warm the area to take away the sting," suggests Evelyn Placek, M.D., a dermatologist in private practice in Scarsdale, New York. Get inside to a warm area and put a washcloth soaked in lukewarm water on your face. "Don't make the water too hot, because that will dry your skin and remove oils from the surface," she says. Then cleanse tender skin with warm water and a rich, gentle product, such as Dove or Oil of Olay liquid cleanser. Wash gently without rubbing. Rinse, and apply petroleum jelly while your skin is still damp.

"A thin coat of petroleum jelly goes a long way," says Dr. Walters. "It's soothing and protective." Apply it two to three times a day.

Seal Away Paper Cuts

"When a letter from a long-time friend or Ed McMahon arrives at my door, I tear it open as fast as I can. Unfortunately, I still haven't won $10,000,000, and I get a lot of paper cuts. Letter openers are a drag, so I just try to be extra careful. But during the wintertime, paper cuts seem unavoidable. Luckily, a friend showed me how to make them go away in no time by taping them with heavy-duty surgical tape."

A paper cut is deceptively tiny, but deep. It throbs and stings so badly that you feel like every nerve ending in your body is centered in your fingertip.

People tend to get paper cuts more frequently in the winter, when dry air and heat sap away skin's natural moisture. "Skin on the hands, especially, becomes dry and rigid, meaning that it's more vulnerable to the paper's sharp edge," says Wilma Bergfeld, M.D., head of clinical research in the department of dermatology at the Cleveland Clinic Foundation.

Because they are superficial, paper cuts heal fast. But they can be very uncomfortable for a few days—especially if you need to use your fingertips, says Dr. Bergfeld. "Every time you move your fingertip, the cut opens again."

Fortunately, healing a paper cut is a cinch. Three quick steps, and you'll hardly notice that it's there.

First, run warm water over the cut to prevent infection. Then, apply a dab of antibacterial ointment, such as Bacitracin, recommends Karen E. Burke, M.D., attending physician at Cabrini Medical Center in

New York City. The ointment will help kill germs, and it also moisturizes the cut so it heals faster.

Finally, close the cut by gently pushing both edges together and applying a small strip of surgical tape, which sticks better than an adhesive bandage. "Position the tape perpendicular to the paper cut so that the cut and the tape form an X. Then pull it tightly across the cut so that the skin will stay together and heal," says Dr. Burke.

Counter Toe Corns with Laces

"I recently purchased a pair of walking shoes that were a tad snug. Two weeks later, I developed painful corns on top of my toes. Luckily, I learned a shoe-lacing technique that gives my toes more room. I lace my sneakers so that one lace goes through the bottom eyelet to the top eyelet on the opposite side. I alternate the other lace through the lace holes. Then, I pull on the single lace, lifting the toe box for more space. After I tried this, the pain disappeared."

Rub your feet the wrong way with the wrong shoes, and they'll respond by growing corns or calluses that can hurt if they grow thick enough to press on nerves.

Lacing narrow shoes in a way that lets your toes breathe is a good idea. But more important is buying shoes that fit in the first place. To size up prospective sneaks, says Nancy Elftman, a certified orthotist/pedorthist (a professional shoe fitter) in La Verne, California, trace your foot on a sheet of paper and take the paper with you when you go shopping. Then place the shoes you are considering on top of the tracing. If any of your foot tracing shows, the shoe is too narrow for your foot.

If corns are a problem for you no matter how perfect a fit, try these interventions to stop the pain.

Soak, then rub. Soften corns or calluses by soaking your feet in plain lukewarm water for 5 to 10 minutes. Then use a pumice stone, available in drugstores, to rub off the dead skin a little at a time.

Note: If you have diabetes, decreased sensation, or decreased circulation, check with a podiatrist before you attempt this, says Cheryl Weiner, D.P.M., president of the American Association for Women Podiatrists.

Oil 'em up. After soaking and rubbing, use a moisturizing cream such as vitamin E cream or vitamin E oil (not vegetable oil) to help keep your feet soft.

Easy Warmup for Cold-Sensitive Hands

"Last winter, I tried downhill skiing for the first time. After a few lessons, I conquered the bunny hill and was ready to hit the slopes—until I developed Raynaud's disease in both hands. When exposed to the cold, my fingers would turn white and hurt so bad that I could no longer ski. Then I discovered hand warmers. Easily tucked into my gloves, the heat pouches kept my fingers warm and pain-free so I could enjoy skiing again."

"We know that Raynaud's is caused by a spasm of the blood vessels," explains Kendra Kaye, M.D., clinical assistant professor of medicine at the University of Pennsylvania School of Medicine in Philadelphia. A glitch in the body's circulatory system triggers a painful, superspastic overreaction to cold that constricts the blood vessels, especially in the fingers and toes.

"What we don't know is why it happens," says Dr. Kaye. But keeping your fingers and toes warm when outdoors is a top priority for someone with Raynaud's. In addition to stocking up on mittens, gloves, and socks, stock up on heat pouches. Available at most department and sports stores, these nifty devices generate heat for six to eight hours after you activate them.

Most strategies to prevent an attack of Raynaud's are focused on temporarily preventing a spasm in the blood vessels. But at the U.S. Army Research Institute of Environmental Medicine in Natick, Massachusetts, researchers are teaching an innovative cold-reconditioning technique. It trains the blood vessels to relax (dilate) rather than constrict when exposed to cold. The submersion technique is somewhat time-consuming, but the results may be worth it. Many people who try it experience remission after only a few repetitions, while others may need to do it 40 to 50 times over several days. For best results, do it in winter when you can use a cold outside area and a warm inside area. Then follow this procedure: Fill two buckets with water of about 100°F. Place one container in a cold area and the other in a warm room. Dressed lightly, in the warm room, immerse both your hands in the water for 2 to 5 minutes. Wrap your hands in a towel and go to the cold area. Again, put your hands in the 100°F water, this time for 10 minutes. Return indoors and put both hands in the 100°F water for 2 to 5 more minutes. Repeat the procedure three to six times a day, every other day.

Healing Moves

Build a Pain-Proof Back

Exercises that strengthen the lower back are good insurance against painful back injuries. A stronger back makes lifting easier as well. Here, Miriam E. Nelson, Ph.D., associate chief of the physiology laboratory at the Jean Mayer U.S. Department of Agriculture Human Nutrition Research Center on Aging at Tufts University in Medford, Massachusetts, and author of Strong Women Stay Slim *and the national bestseller* Strong Women Stay Young, *presents a lower-back exercise, with tips to keep from injuring your back while exercising.*

Given a choice, you're probably more likely to exercise your arms and legs than your lower back. Who can blame you? Every time you look in a mirror, you get to admire the results of your hard work. Your back, on the other hand, often goes unnoticed.

Despite minimum exposure, there are lots of good reasons to stop overlooking the back extensor muscles. Most important, strong lower-back muscles are the best shield against agonizing back pain and injury.

Plus, it will be easier to lift heavy suitcases and grocery bags, you'll stand taller, and activities like tennis, golf, gardening, and skiing will be a whole lot easier to do. If that isn't enough motivation, invest in a three-way mirror. You'll see the results in six to eight weeks.

Each lift should last three seconds, with a three-second pause and three seconds to lower—keeping your breath easy and natural the whole time. Eight to 12 extensions is considered a set. Do one to three sets, two to three sessions per week, and allow at least one day of rest between workouts.

If you can't do 8 repetitions, the effort is too much. For an easier version, use partial movements. For example, lift only halfway. When you can easily do 12 repetitions, the effort is too little, and you need to move to the more advanced versions.

As you're trying this exercise, keep these very important pointers in mind: Don't arch your back excessively or lift your arms higher than the rest of your body. And remember to move slowly through the exercise.

If you have a bad back or have had a back injury in the past, check with your doctor before trying this exercise.

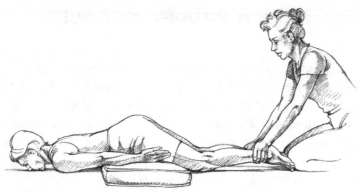

Have a partner hold your ankles. Position your hips about five to six inches off the floor (place pillows under your pelvis). Turn your palms to face your thighs. Keep your arms straight along the sides of your body. Lie face down.

No partner? Tuck your feet under a sturdy piece of furniture or don a pair of ankle weights (about 15 pounds each) to help hold your legs down.

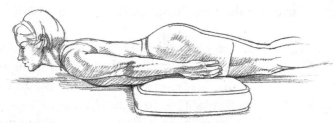

Using your lower-back muscles, slowly lift your head, trunk, and chest off the floor. Come up only as far as you feel comfortable.

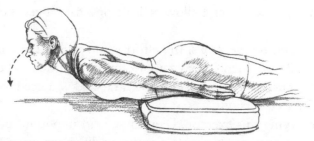

Ultimately, you should continue lifting until your upper body is in line with your legs. Hold, and then slowly lower.

Wipe Away Lower-Back Fatigue

Twenty minutes after sliding behind the wheel, your back starts to announce each passing mile. Luckily, there's a simple way to soothe these twinges after car trips—or whenever you've been sitting still too long. It's called the Windshield Wiper.

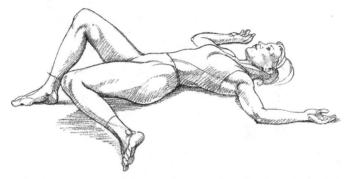

Wipe in. Keeping one leg upright, gently drop the other knee in and down as far as you can, rolling onto the inside of your foot. Try to keep that side of your pelvis on the ground. It's okay if it comes off slightly, though. Gently press your buttocks bones down so that your lower back arches up slightly. Then tuck your tailbone forward and extend your leg from pelvis to knee. Hold and breathe softly for 30 seconds.

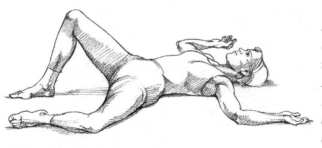

Wipe out. Drop your knee to the outside, letting the other leg fall inward if needed. Hold and breathe for 30 seconds. Wipe in and out twice with each leg.

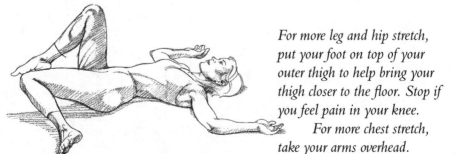

For more leg and hip stretch, put your foot on top of your outer thigh to help bring your thigh closer to the floor. Stop if you feel pain in your knee.
For more chest stretch, take your arms overhead.

part 7

Achieving Optimum Health: A Woman's Guide

Making Sense of It All

There's no better time to be a woman. With all the new women's health research—in nutrition, fitness, medicine, and, of course, natural healing—we can raise the bar on our health expectations. Yes, we can live longer and better than any generation before . . . if we take action now.

Do you know what your cholesterol number is? You should. That simple blood test is as important as an annual mammogram. That's because heart disease is women's health enemy number one. It claims more women's lives than any other disease, including breast cancer. But if you nab the problem early enough, you can take gender-specific steps to protect yourself.

And there's more encouraging news for women: The stereotypical elder lady who's small, stooped, frail, and fearful of breaking her hip is becoming extinct. By taking the right steps now to maintain good, healthy bones, women today can forever walk tall with perfect posture and strong, healthy gaits. The secret is in our lifestyle—with a little help from medical science.

Menopause, of course, continues to offer challenges aplenty for us just as it did for our mothers. The difference is, we have more options available to help us ease through it. Just look what has happened to hormone replacement therapy. It has gone from one-size-fits-all to an amazing, expanding array of pills, patches, and creams in dozens of new formulas and doses. Or, if you prefer to go all-natural, science gives a cool thumbs-up to certain herbs, foods, and vitamin supplements for "the change."

Speaking of natural remedies, you'll find others here to help you overcome those common female complaints like yeast infections, urinary incontinence, and morning sickness. And read about the latest preventive advice for breast and endometrial (uterine) cancers.

So, if you're determined to look younger, feel stronger, and live longer than any generation before, here's the year's top tools and expert advice to help you achieve your goals.

Positive Action Plans

A Heart-Smart Guide to Living Longer: What Every Woman Must Know

Nancy Beall had a heart attack in 1996 and didn't know it. "I sat up all night long," says the 57-year-old Baltimore administrative assistant. "It was like all the muscles in my body felt tired and weak. All my joints hurt. I thought, 'Gosh, maybe I have rheumatoid arthritis!' I had achiness in my arms. But there was nothing that I would call pain."

Early in the morning, she called the cardiologist who had been caring for her for years. "He just happened to be in his office at 7:00 A.M., standing by the phone. He told me to go straight to the emergency room. He ordered me to tell the attending doctor that I have atypical symptoms and to consult with him while waiting for the results."

Immediately, Beall called an ambulance and went to the hospital. The emergency room doctors did two cardiac enzyme tests, which showed no sign of heart attack. They told her that she had a flu and wanted to send her home. "But my daughter kept insisting they do the test again. She kept repeating that my symptoms were atypical." Sure enough, the third enzyme test showed that she had really had a heart attack.

"It turned out that three of my four heart arteries were 99 percent occluded." To remove the occlusion—or blockage—doctors needed to act right away. Beall's life was saved by an immediate quadruple bypass.

Like the emergency room doctors, many people still think of heart attacks as a man's problem. The truth is that heart disease kills more women every year than do all forms of cancer, chronic lung disease, pneumonia, diabetes, accidents, and AIDS combined. That's more than half a million women.

And it's not just women who underestimate their risk. Even some doctors still think of heart disease as primarily a man's problem. Studies have found that doctors provide women with less testing, less follow-up, less treatment, and less surgery.

That may partly explain why, once heart disease does strike, it's far deadlier for women. Women are more than 1½ times as likely to die within a year of their first heart attack than are men.

Here is what women need to know about the risk factors, symptoms, new testing devices, and an important new link between heart disease and depression.

Diagnosing Heart Disease

Great technology for diagnosing heart disease in men has been around for a long time. One test is the treadmill stress test, when an ECG (electrocardiogram) is performed continuously during exercise. This test works fine for men, but in women it produces false positives (indicating that there is a heart problem when there really isn't) more than a third of the time and false negatives (indicating no problem when there really is one) about a fourth of the time.

"Women's survival was being harmed," says D. Douglas Miller, M.D., professor of internal medicine and medical director of the Cardiac Stress Laboratory at St. Louis University. Some women who really didn't have heart disease were sent on for unnecessary and invasive tests. Or some doctors decided to ignore the stress ECG results that showed a problem, betting that the woman was really fine and the machine was wrong. Studies show that after a positive ECG, women are not as likely as men to be followed up with subsequent testing.

Over the past 5 to 10 years, a great deal of effort has been directed toward gender-equivalent testing. "We're now at a point where equivalence is virtually achieved," says Dr. Miller.

The two most accurate new techniques involve imaging. "Whenever possible, these are the tests that a woman should ask for," says Rita Redberg, M.D., associate professor of medicine at the University of California in San Francisco and a member of the American Heart Association Council on Clinical Cardiology.

The first of these new imaging techniques involves having a patient walk on a treadmill, then injecting a radioactive isotope (known as technetium 99 sestamibi) into the bloodstream, which allows special scanners to track the blood flow through the heart.

Another option is the stress echocardiogram test. Cardiologist and *Prevention* advisor Marianne Legato, M.D., director of Partnership for

Women's Health at Columbia University in New York City, prefers it because there's no injection, it's accurate, sensitive, and less expensive, and it doesn't take as long as the technetium test.

Not all imaging tests, however, are as good. A far less accurate option is the thallium 201 radioisotope test, which was developed for men but doesn't work as well in women.

Who should get tested? Experts agree that the stress echocardiogram or technetium tests are usually not necessary for women before menopause who have no risk factors for heart disease.

Women who have symptoms or strong risk factors should get tested, Dr. Legato explains. "I reserve the tests for women who have some concern for heart disease risk—perhaps they have new pains, they smoke, they're sedentary, they have family histories of diabetes, or they have diabetes." She recommends testing at least annually for women with symptoms.

If you're going to have a test, Dr. Miller says, it's a good idea to find out what kind. If stress ECG or thallium imaging are your only choices, they're better than nothing, but make sure that you follow up with your doctor and ask for retesting if the first test suggests there's a problem.

Women's Symptoms: Different, but Just as Deadly

What does a heart attack feel like?

For men, it's often the classic chest-clutching pain, tightness, or heaviness in the chest, usually accompanied by shortness of breath or sweating.

For women, a heart attack can be competely different. Women may experience little or no chest pain, says cardiologist Roy Ziegelstein, M.D., deputy chairman of the department of medicine at the Johns Hopkins Bayview Medical Center in Baltimore. Because the symptoms may be so unlike a typical male heart attack, female symptoms may be described as atypical.

During a heart attack, women often experience shortness of breath or difficulty breathing and may even have pain or weakness in the shoulders, arms, or all over the body. Women are more likely than men to experience what feels like nausea, which is not relieved by antacids or burping. There may even be vomiting. The symptoms are more likely to

(continued on page 224)

Reducing Your Risk

"The risk factors in women are pretty much the same as they are in men," says John C. LaRosa, M.D., chancellor at Tulane University Medical Center in New Orleans and a member of the American Heart Association Risk Factors Task Force. "But there are some subtle differences." It's important to know what they are. Here's a review of the major heart disease risk factors and what you can do about them.

Risk factor: smoking. Women who smoke heavily increase their heart disease risk two to four times.

What to do: Quit. It works. After smoking cessation, risk in both women and men tumbles within months, and within three to five years is as low as the risk for nonsmokers.

Risk factor: high cholesterol. For men or women with total cholesterol below 150 mg/dl (milligrams per deciliter), it is very difficult to get heart disease. With more than 150 mg/dl, both men and women are more susceptible, and the higher it goes, the more susceptible they are. But important differences between the genders do exist.

Men can generally use their total cholesterol to tell whether they're at risk. But women need to break the total down and learn their "good" HDL (high-density lipoprotein) and "bad" LDL (low-density lipoprotein) numbers. Then, they should divide the total by the HDL. The result is called the total/HDL ratio. The goal is to be at 4.0 or lower. Anything more than that means an elevated risk of heart disease.

What to do: Regular exercise and a diet that's low in total fat and animal fats can lower LDLs and reduce overall cholesterol.

Risk factor: high blood pressure. For both men and women, target blood pressure should be 130 systolic (top) and 85 diastolic (bottom). If either number is higher, it may mean an increased risk of heart disease.

What to do: Have your blood pressure checked at least every 2½ years. Treating and controlling high blood pressure can reduce heart disease risk significantly.

Risk factor: physical inactivity. Physically active women have a 60 to 75 percent lower risk of heart disease than inactive women do.

What to do: With your doctor's okay, walk two miles a day or get the equivalent in another form of exercise.

Risk factor: diabetes. Regardless of her age, a woman with diabetes has the same risk of heart disease as a man does and a risk three to seven times higher than that of a woman without diabetes.

What to do: Maintain a healthy weight, stay active, and reduce dietary fat intake to help delay and control diabetes.

Risk factor: waist/hip ratio. Both obesity and a high waist/hip ratio are risk factors for heart disease. A high waist/hip ratio usually signifies too much fat on the abdomen.

To determine your waist/hip ratio, take the measurement of your waist and divide it by the measurement of your hips. The target number is 0.8 or below. Above 0.8, research shows that the risk of heart disease rises steeply in women. For example, if your waist is 27 inches and your hips measure 34 inches, your waist/hip ratio is 0.79, so you're on the safe side.

What to do: Lose a little weight. The good news is that it's not so hard to change a waist/hip ratio by losing a little weight. Even five pounds lost can make the difference.

Risk factor: high triglycerides. High triglycerides are more powerful predictors of risk in women than in men, especially after women reach age 50. "Triglycerides are not cholesterol, but they're a marker for the same carriers that bring cholesterol to the blood vessel wall," explains Dr. LaRosa. "Anything more than 150 begins to accelerate the uptake of cholesterol into the blood vessel wall."

What to do: Weight loss, even as little as 15 pounds around the waist, can reduce triglycerides.

Risk factor: age. Men's risk of heart attack and stroke soars after age 45. In women, the risk rises when they're about 10 years older. Researchers believe that the gradual drop in estrogen after menopause may be partly responsible.

What to do: While there's not much you can do about your age, there is research suggesting that estrogen replacement therapy can significantly reduce postmenopausal women's heart disease risk.

Risk factor: family history and race. A family history of heart disease is even more common in women with coronary heart disease than in men. Your risk of heart disease or stroke is higher if a close family member had any of these diseases. Race makes a difference too: African-Americans have a higher risk than Caucasian Americans do, partly because of a tendency toward high blood pressure.

What to do: Adopt heart-healthy habits and get regular and complete checkups. African-Americans, and everyone with a family history, should be particularly vigilant.

occur when women are resting, or during mental stress or physical exercise. Women are also likely to experience fatigue. "Not, 'I fall asleep at 5:00 P.M. every night' fatigue," Dr. Ziegelstein explains, "but feeling completely wiped out." Dr. Ziegelstein also cites "a general sense of being unwell; that something really wrong is going on."

In women, atypical symptoms may come and go, signifying angina (a temporary lack of oxygen to the heart, which can be a warning sign of a future heart attack). When they occur at the beginning of a heart attack, symptoms usually don't go away, and they can become worse as minutes or hours pass.

Time Is Muscle: What to Do

Assume that you're experiencing some of these feelings—say, extreme exhaustion, shoulder and arm pain, fatigue. Something's wrong. Could be flu or a heart attack. How can you tell?

"You can't," says Irving Kron, M.D., chief of cardiothoracic surgery at the University of Virginia Medical Center in Charlottesville and vice chairman of the American Heart Association Council on Cardiovascular Surgery. "You have something that gets you nervous? Get it checked out."

And do it fast. "Time is muscle," says Dr. Miller. Don't delay. Here's what to do.

Call your doctor. If you can't reach your doctor, make sure you let the person on the other end know that you believe it's a medical emergency.

Chew an aspirin. "Chewing a 325-milligram aspirin in the early stages of a heart attack has been shown to improve the rate of survival in men and women," says Dr. Miller.

Head for the emergency room. Do this if the symptoms are extreme, and have the medical staff or a family member alert your physician.

Don't worry about your potential embarrassment if you're wrong and you really do have the flu. Studies show that women tend to delay much longer than men do before showing up at a hospital with a heart attack—as much as four hours longer. "Women and men both have to be willing to feel foolish," says Dr. Kron. "Your chances of surviving, if it is a heart attack, are much better if you're at the hospital than if you're at home wondering."

And when you're describing symptoms to any doctor, be as specific as possible, adds Dr. Legato. "Don't say, 'I have a funny feeling.' Say, 'I have chest discomfort when I am upset. It is a burning pain that goes to my neck and shoulders.'"

Depression: Women Must Pay Attention

For both men and women, says *Prevention* advisor Redford B. Williams, M.D., professor of psychiatry and director of the Behavioral Medicine Research Center at Duke University School of Medicine in Durham, North Carolina, the latest studies link three psychosocial risk factors to a higher risk and worse prognosis for heart disease. They are hostility, social isolation, and depression.

As Dr. Williams explains, men are more likely to have hostility and less likely to have social support. Women tend to have more social support and—as a group—they tend to display less hostility than men. But women are also twice as likely to experience depression.

Could depression be one factor explaining why heart disease kills as many women as it does men? Nancy Frasure-Smith, Ph.D., associate professor of psychiatry and nursing at Montreal University, tracked 613 men and 283 women who'd had heart attacks. "We found that people who were depressed—men or women—were three to four times more likely to die of cardiac causes. That makes depression as dangerous to the heart as traditional risk factors like high blood pressure or smoking."

How might depression harm the heart? Dr. Ziegelstein, who did a similar study of depression and mortality in more than 200 male and female heart attack patients, offers some theories.

"We found that patients who were depressed had lower adherence to a risk-reduction program," says Dr. Ziegelstein. "Depressed people often lose interest in helping themselves." Another possible explanation, says Dr. Ziegelstein, is a link between the heart and the brain. "The damaging processes may be tied to the level of serotonin in the brain, which may make them more apt to develop a fatal rhythm abnormality."

Whatever the cause, experts agree, research suggests that pervasive sadness after a heart attack should be addressed and treated promptly.

"A lot of people think that very mild depression after a heart attack is perfectly normal and will go away by itself," says Dr. Ziegelstein. "And in many instances, they're correct. But if it doesn't go away, it should be cause for concern."

In particular, alarms should go off if the depression is very deep or lasts

Resources for Heart Healing

Heart disease is a challenge that you don't want to face alone . . . if you can help it. Here are some organizations that can help provide support.

Mended Hearts. A national organization with more than 260 chapters across the United States, offering information and support for people who have heart disease as well as for their families and friends. Find the nearest chapter by writing to Mended Hearts, 7272 Greenville Avenue, Dallas, TX 75231-4596.

Depressed Anonymous. An international 12-step organization inspired by a woman who suffered from heart disease and depression. Offers local support groups for depression. For free information, send a self-addressed stamped envelope to Depressed Anonymous, P.O. Box 17471, Louisville, KY 40217.

Emotions Anonymous. An international organization with more than 1,000 chapters. Fellowship for people experiencing emotional difficulties. Uses the 12-step program, sharing experiences, strength, and hopes in order to improve emotional health. Correspondence program for those who cannot attend meetings. Contact Emotions Anonymous, P.O. Box 4245, St. Paul, MN 55104-0245.

longer than a month. "Even milder forms of sadness that go on for longer than a month after a heart attack need attention," says Dr. Ziegelstein.

He notes that, in some cases, mild depression could be a reaction to medication, and the patient may need the doctor to make an adjustment. (Never stop taking heart medication without consulting your physician.) Or it may be that the person needs additional psychological and emotional help. It's critical to raise the issue with your doctor. "And if the doctor doesn't respond," says Dr. Ziegelstein, "get a new doctor or ask for a referral to a psychiatrist or a psychologist."

What are the best treatments for depression after heart attack? Experts cite one powerful weapon that is available in virtually every hospital in the country: the cardiac rehabilitation group.

Barbara Riegel, D.N.Sc. (doctor of nursing science), a cardiovascular researcher and associate professor of nursing at the San Diego State University School of Nursing, notes, "Good cardiac rehabilitation groups include a lot of components: exercise, useful information classes, and emotional support." Some groups offer other healing therapies, she adds. "They may bring in components of meditation, stress reduction, and behavioral psychology."

If a group isn't available, there are other options, says Dr. Riegel. "Activate your social support system; just be around other people." (There are also some wonderful nationally based support groups for heart patients and for anyone with depression.

Individual counseling and cognitive and behavioral therapy, which are well-proven to combat depression in healthy people, may be an appropriate route for heart patients.

Antidepressant medications for heart patients are more controversial. "Some patients would benefit from antidepressant medication," says Dr. Ziegelstein. "But someone who has had a heart attack is on a lot of other medications, and there are concerns about drug interactions as well as toxicity to damaged hearts. There isn't enough research to be sure." Ideally, a heart patient on antidepressants should be under the care of (or in consultation with) an experienced psychiatrist or psychopharmacologist.

What about depression in women who don't have heart disease? Can dealing with depression reduce their chances of ever getting heart disease? Dr. Legato is convinced that the answer is yes. "All my patients have reported, 'I was so stressed the month before my heart attack.' My experience is that the kind of emotional pain that people who develop heart disease are suffering is the kind for which they have no answer, no possible escape."

To ease the pain, Dr. Legato says, everyone should seek out a confidante, whether it's a doctor, friend, or relative. "Everyone needs someone to whom she can lay out her problems. Many times, just verbalizing will begin a train of thought that produces a solution."

Is Your Estrogen Giving You What You Want?

If you could take all the estrogen products that are available and line them up on one shelf, you might think that you were in the cereal aisle of your supermarket. The sheer variety is overwhelming.

First, there are all the different types of estrogen. You practically need a degree in pharmacology to pronounce their names, let alone understand the chemical differences between them: estradiol, conjugated estrogens, estropipate, esterified estrogen, and estrone. What's more, estrogens come in a variety of delivery systems: pills, transdermal patches, creams, and even a new intravaginal ring. And most of these products come in different dosages.

How do you know what's right for you? True, all forms of estrogen replacement therapy are intended to ease menopause in one way or another. They may stop what are called vasomotor symptoms—symptoms like hot flashes and night sweats. Or quench symptoms of urogenital atrophy: vaginal dryness, painful intercourse, and urinary tract discomforts. Or halt bone loss that can lead to crippling osteoporosis. And there's even the tantalizing, albeit preliminary, evidence that estrogen supplementation may halve a woman's risk of heart disease.

Thinking that there's one perfect estrogen for everyone is like suggesting to every cereal-lover in the supermarket that they only buy a big white box marked "Breakfast Flakes." The point is, there's no single perfect estrogen, and not every estrogen does it all.

The woman who switches to the patch because a pill has made her queasy also has to say good-bye to the rise in heart-healthy HDL that can come with the pill. And she may find that she has skin irritation from the patch. A switch in any direction has its trade-offs, and some trades are more serious than others.

What to do? Prioritize, says Howard Zacur, M.D., Ph.D., professor of reproductive endocrinology and director of the estrogen consultation service at Johns Hopkins Medical Institutions in Baltimore. "List your goals in order of importance to you, whether it's relief of vasomotor symptoms or something bigger, like bone protection." If you're not sure, a complete physical examination and a cholesterol test can determine whether cardiovascular protection is an urgent need for you. A bone density test can help you figure out whether bone protection should be a top concern, or—if you're already on estrogen—whether it is helping your bones enough.

Look for your number one priority below, and find which form of estrogen can give it to you.

Priority: Relief from Dryness

Without adequate amounts of estrogen, the tissues in the vagina and urinary tract become dry, atrophied, and easily traumatized. Vaginal dryness can cause painful intercourse as well as uncomfortable itching. Many women also experience increases in urinary tract infections and irritation of the urethra, which can cause painful urination.

If these annoying and persistent complaints are your only reason to take estrogen replacement therapy, a localized form of estrogen, supplied by prescription vaginal estrogen creams or the new vaginal ring, may be all you need.

The down side is that localized estrogen doesn't prevent hot flashes or help your heart or bones. "If someone came to me saying, 'I want to prevent heart disease,' I would not advise her to use a vaginal cream," says Valerie L. Baker, M.D., gynecologist and reproductive endocrinologist at the University of California, San Francisco. Nor would the ring be the way to go.

If you're looking to get the added benefits of relief from hot flashes and night sweats and protection against bone loss or heart disease (which looks promising but not yet proven), you'll need the pill or patch form of estrogen.

Vaginal creams are applied directly into the vagina. Depending on whom you ask, that's a blessing—or a mess.

Creams, however, may be a quick way to combat vaginal dryness, which is the only thing they are intended to do. While it can take a month to get relief through a pill or patch, creams may bring relief slightly faster (the vaginal tissues absorb them very well). Creams, used as prescribed, also don't elevate blood levels of estrogen significantly or consistently, because the estrogen really stays mostly in the vagina, says Brian Walsh, M.D., director of the menopause clinic at Brigham and Women's Hospital in Boston.

If you use the cream sporadically or find success with smaller amounts than those recommended on the package, you may have even smaller amounts of estrogen circulating in your body.

Vaginal rings were first designed for contraception. But earlier this year, Estring became available in the United States for estrogen replacement therapy. About the size of a diaphragm, it is inserted by either the woman or her physician and kept for up to three months in the vagina, where it releases a steady, low dose of estrogen. Clinical studies show that it works well to relieve both vaginal dryness and urinary tract complaints. It may be more convenient and certainly less messy than creams. And unlike creams, you don't have to think about when to apply it.

"The ring is specifically designed to deliver estrogen locally and in doses too low to provide blood levels of estrogen comparable to the patch or pill. So very minimal levels get into the blood," says Dr. Zacur. Like the creams, the ring won't provide relief from hot flashes or a benefit to your bones or heart.

Priority: Relief from Hot Flashes

When the body lacks adequate levels of estrogen, it tricks the brain into thinking that your body's temperature is too high. As a result, blood flow increases to your skin, you become overheated and flushed, and you begin to perspire. If taming hot flashes or night sweats is your number one goal, your only choices are an estrogen taken orally or the transdermal patch, because nothing else gets enough estrogen to the temperature regulation center in the brain.

If doctors tend to prescribe the pill called Premarin more frequently, it's most likely because of all the studies on it. "Because it's the most widely tested estrogen, I think that it's worth considering if a woman chooses oral estrogen," says Nanette Santoro, M.D., associate professor in the department of obstetrics and gynecology at the UMDNJD–New Jersey Medical School in Newark.

Nonetheless, the patch can also relieve hot flashes and night sweats. The patch is self-adhesive and releases estrogen through the skin into the bloodstream. It is applied to the buttocks or abdomen, according to the manufacturer's instructions, and changed once or twice a week (depending on the brand you choose).

If you haven't decided between the pill or patch, turn to your next priority—maybe heart or bone protection—to give you a hand. See those sections for insights that can help you make your decision.

Keep in mind that if you're set on relieving hot flashes and night sweats, there may be some nonestrogen ways to do that, such as by eating foods containing soy.

Priority: Bone Protection

If one of your priorities for estrogen is that it protects your bones, know that several oral estrogens—at certain doses—and one transdermal patch are indicated by the Food and Drug Administration (FDA) for preventing bone loss. Other patches and pills are likely to follow as the manufacturers do the necessary studies to convince the FDA of the bone-protecting abilities.

With bone protection, the biggest point seems to be dosage. Go too low and your bones get no benefit. The challenge? There's no magic cutoff point (yet) under which bones are not being helped. Each product has to show efficacy on its own. So far, here's what has been shown to benefit bone.

The minimum bone-protecting dose approved by the FDA for oral estrogens is 0.5 milligram of Estrace, 0.75 milligram of Ogen, 0.75 milligram of Ortho-Est, and 0.625 milligram of Premarin. In the estrogen patch category, the FDA has approved Estraderm at 0.05 milligram.

Even if a product is FDA-approved for osteoporosis prevention at only one dose, that doesn't mean a physician can't prescribe a higher dose. In fact, a some experts feel that some of the approved doses are too low for maximum bone protection.

If you see that the dose you're currently taking may not be high enough for bone benefits, you have a couple of choices. One, of course, is to ask your doctor about taking more estrogen. But remember: There are risks and benefits to be balanced.

Estrogen isn't the only medication that can halt bone loss either. Another option is alendronate.

Also, make sure that you're getting plenty of vitamin D, from daily outings in sunshine or from milk or multivitamins. Remember, too, that you still need your 1,500 milligrams of calcium daily even when you're taking estrogen. And don't forget regular weight-bearing exercise. Don't smoke. Decrease your drinking. While none of these actions, by itself, can halt bone loss, there's a cumulative effect if you enforce the habits that tend to build bone and decrease the habits that can contribute to bone loss. "All of these may be additive," says Bruce Carr, M.D., director of the division of reproductive endocrinology at the University of Texas Southwestern Medical Center in Dallas.

Priority: Heart Protection

If heart disease protection tops your list of reasons to take estrogen, both the pill and the patch have benefits to offer. But the benefits of each are slightly different.

If crunching of your cholesterol numbers is what the doctor or-

What's Become of Estrogen Risk?

As doctors began prescribing hormone replacement therapy for women, researchers began reporting the incidence of certain kinds of cancer. Here are their conclusions to date.

Endometrial cancer. Taking estrogen in either a pill or patch stimulates the cells of the endometrium (lining of the uterus) to grow and thicken. If this growth is excessive, and goes undetected and untreated, it can be an early step in the development of cancer.

It has become standard for women to take a progestogen along with their pill or patch. (The exception is women who have had hysterectomies: Because their uteruses have been removed, there's no risk of cancer.) Its job is to trigger the uterine lining to stop growing and to shed periodically. Some women would rather do without the bleeding, but physicians can say with certainty that it wards off the increased risk.

What about vaginal estrogen creams? Exceeding the recommended doses of the cream might well increase estrogen levels to a point comparable to the patch or pill. "Endometrial cancer can happen to women who use cream," says Nanette Santoro, M.D., associate professor in the department of obstetrics and gynecology at the UMDNJD–New Jersey Medical School in Newark. She adds that women who use estrogen cream twice a week or more for more than a few months should talk with their doctors about taking a progestogen.

Women have also wondered about the newly introduced vaginal ring that provides a localized form of estrogen. The clinical studies presented to the Food and Drug Administration show that the vaginal ring

dered, then oral estrogens may offer the most powerful heart protection. Because the pill requires digestion, it passes through the liver. This so-called first-pass effect is responsible for increasing the good HDL (high-density lipoprotein) cholesterol and decreasing the bad LDL (low-density lipoprotein) cholesterol.

"If you're looking for major lipid changes, you need to take your estrogen orally," says Dr. Walsh. "The changes are significant. We're talking about a 15 percent increase in HDL. From that alone, you could expect it could reduce heart disease risk something on the order of 40 percent." (Keep in mind that while population studies link estrogen to heart disease prevention, well-controlled trials to prove the point are still

causes very minimal changes in the endometrium and that a progestogen is probably not needed. But since there is limited experience with the ring, compared with pills and patches, it may be best to err on the side of caution. A women using it needs to have her endometrium monitored by her physician to be on the safe side.

Breast cancer. This is the biggie. Oral estrogen taken for long stretches may be associated with an increased risk of breast cancer. How much estrogen, you ask? Unfortunately, scientists can't say with certainty yet whether there's a safe dose or range of doses of estrogen that will not increase breast cancer. "In general, there is concern that the more estrogen you take, and the longer you take it, the greater the risk of breast cancer," says Dr. Santoro.

Regarding the patch, "I would say that the risk of breast cancer from the patch is the same as for oral estrogen, with one caveat," says Brian Walsh, M.D., director of the menopause clinic at Brigham and Women's Hospital in Boston. "Our experience with patches is not as long as with oral. No one has done a head-to-head comparison of the two forms and cancer rates. So we don't know for sure."

The good news about the creams, Dr. Walsh says, is that you're not likely to increase breast cancer risk at all, as long as the creams are not overused. "If I have a patient whose major complaint is vaginal dryness, and she doesn't want to take estrogen, because her sister had breast cancer, that's the kind of woman it's ideal for."

According to experts, the ring is unlikely to increase the risk of breast cancer because it is delivering estrogen locally, at a very low dose.

under way. So at this point, no estrogen has FDA approval for heart protection.)

As far as dose goes, "the level of estrogen needed for the heart is probably comparable to the level needed to protect bones," says Dr. Carr. "But there isn't enough research to be specific yet."

Now the downside: Oral estrogens can raise triglyceride levels (again, the first-pass effect at work). Women who have had blood clots or who are at risk for them and who have gallbladder disease should discuss with their doctors the decision to take oral estrogens. If you're looking for less of an effect on your cholesterol, the patch could help you out. Overall, the patch may come in second place (after pills) for cardiovascular benefits, but that's still pretty good. Although oral estrogens have the most beneficial effect on cholesterol levels, research shows that estrogen from patch as well as pill has a direct benefit on blood vessels—improving blood flow, for example. "In the long run, the benefits via direct action on the blood vessels may be as helpful in preventing heart disease as estrogen's effect on cholesterol," says Dr. Baker.

Unlike oral estrogens, the patch doesn't increase triglycerides. Even though studies aren't conclusive, it is likely to have minimal or no effect on blood clotting. So it's considered safe for women who can't take pills for those reasons, though any decision like this should be discussed with your doctor.

Of course, when it comes to protecting the heart, there are ways to do it in addition to estrogen therapy: Eat a low-fat diet, exercise, reduce stress, and of course, don't smoke.

Read This before You Say Yes to Hysterectomy

The numbers are staggering. Each year, more than half a million women undergo hysterectomies, the second most common surgery in America among women of reproductive age. And it's major surgery. Recovery can take weeks or months, and as with any surgery, there's a real risk of death—an estimated 1 in 1,000 women die from this procedure.

In short, it's no small thing, and it's usually unnecessary. "About 90 percent of women who have hysterectomies could have been offered an alternative," says Brian Walsh, M.D., director of the menopause clinic at Brigham and Women's Hospital in Boston. But most women are never given the choice.

Why? Some doctors don't know about the options. Today, there are safer alternatives. Virtually all involve fewer risks, less bloodshed, and a shorter (or no) recovery time. And some doctors don't mention procedures that they don't have the skills to perform themselves.

So what do you do when your doctor tells you that you need a hysterectomy? Here are three of the most common causes of hysterectomy and the ways to treat them that don't involve removing your uterus.

Fibroids

What are they? Fibroids, or uterine leiomyomas, are bundles of muscle and connective tissue that can grow inside or outside the uterus. Not much is known about why they start, says Adriane Fugh-Berman, M.D., chairwoman of the National Women's Health Network, an independent consumer advocacy organization in Washington, D.C.; a nationally recognized authority on alternative medicine; and author of *Alternative Medicine: What Works.* "We do know that estrogen makes them grow. And that when women go through menopause, fibroids usually shrink, unless women take hormone replacement therapy (HRT)." Fibroids are virtually always benign. But they're the number one cause of hysterectomy (prompting a third of all hysterectomy surgeries in the United States).

How common are they? About a quarter of all women in their thirties and forties could have fibroids.

What are the symptoms? As fibroids grow, they are more likely to trigger symptoms that are not life-threatening, but that can sometimes make life miserable. "They can cause bleeding—in some cases, heavy bleeding throughout the menstrual cycle—leading to anemia," notes Dr. Walsh. Other symptoms include pain, frequent urination, infertility, and recurrent miscarriages.

How are they best diagnosed? Along with a complete history and thorough pelvic examination, the doctor should perform two kinds of ultrasound: an abdominal ultrasound, done from the top of the belly, to rule out the possibility of ovarian cancer; and transvaginal ultrasound, done by inserting a probe inside the vagina, to pinpoint the exact size and location of the fibroids. These are simple office procedures that don't require an incision or anesthesia.

What are the treatment alternatives?

Watching and waiting. "Sometimes, I've counseled women who may be fairly close to menopause to just wait," says Dr. Fugh-Berman.

But it is a good idea to have fibroids checked regularly by a physician to make sure that they're not growing rapidly. Check every six months when the fibroids first appear.

After six months, says Dr. Walsh, "if a fibroid has only grown from two inches to three inches, that's not fast, and you can stretch out checkups to annually. If it has grown from two inches to eight inches, that's cause for concern." Another danger sign is when new fibroids appear or

Your Resources
for Hysterectomy Research

Your doctor says you need a hysterectomy. You're not so sure. What do you say? Michael E. Toaff, M.D., senior attending physician at Bryn Mawr Hospital in Pennsylvania, has this to say: "Ask, 'Is there any procedure, short of hysterectomy, either medical or surgical, that could resolve my problem?'"

If you don't get a satisfactory answer, where do you turn next? Your top priority, experts agree, should be to find a physician or surgeon who is experienced in the alternatives you are considering. How?

Try a teaching hospital for a second opinion or treatment. A Canadian study showed that health care providers who are affiliated with teaching hospitals perform hysterectomy less often than providers who are not affiliated with teaching hospitals. "They have access to the latest medical technology and research," says Howard A. Zacur, M.D., Ph.D., professor of reproductive endocrinology and director of the estrogen consultation service at Johns Hopkins Medical Institutions in Baltimore.

Or, contact HERS (Hysterectomy Educational Resources and Services). This pioneering organization located in Bala Cynwyd, Pennsylvania, is an invaluable resource for women determined to keep their uterus. "We counsel each woman individually and tell her what her options are depending on her history," says Nora Coffey, director. Counseling is a reasonable $10 an hour. Contact HERS 422 Bryn Mawr Avenue, Bala Cynwyd, PA 19004. HERS can also provide names of skilled physicians in your region.

If you have fibroids, get a great doctor. "Just because she has done tons of hysterectomies, that doesn't qualify her to do myomectomy (removal of fibroids, leaving the uterus intact)," points out Adriane Fugh-Berman, M.D., chairwoman of the National Women's Health Network, an

rapid fibroid growth occurs in women who are past menopause (even women on HRT).

Nonsteroidal anti-inflammatories (NSAIDs), such as Motrin, can sometimes help ease the pain and heavy bleeding from fibroids.

Myomectomy. This surgery removes the fibroids, leaving the uterus

independent consumer advocacy organization in Washington, D.C.; a nationally recognized authority on alternative medicine; and author of *Alternative Medicine: What Works*. "It's a difficult procedure and takes a longer time to learn." Here are questions you should ask the doctor you're considering.

• Do you ever give a transfusion during a myomectomy? "The correct answer is no. If the answer is that most women need a blood transfusion, then you're in the wrong office," says Coffey.

Dr. Toaff adds, "I haven't given one in the last 250 procedures that I've done. If the doctor has great expertise, it's very, very rare that he has to give the patient blood."

• Are you board certified in gynecology? The correct answer is yes.

• How many myomectomies have you performed? The correct answer, says Dr. Toaff, should be in the hundreds. How many have you done in the past year? "At least 50 cases a year," says Dr. Toaff, "so they have real ongoing experience."

• How many surgeries that started as myomectomies ended up as hysterectomies? "If it's more than 2 percent, it's too many," says Coffey.

• Have you done many surgeries for fibroids as large as mine? The best answer is yes, plenty.

If you have endometriosis, contact the Endometriosis Association, headquartered in Milwaukee. This international self-help organization offers many valuable resources. For information, write to the Endometriosis Association at 8585 North 76th Place, Milwaukee, WI 53223.

A must-have book is the *Endometriosis Sourcebook* by Mary Lou Ballweg and the Endometriosis Association. This book offers the latest information on endometriosis and is available in bookstores as well as from the Endometriosis Association. The book describes conventional and alternative treatments and includes an extensive discussion of the pros and cons of hysterectomy.

intact. Myomectomies are becoming more routine outside of Europe. An estimated 123,000 U.S. women choose them every year, but it still can take an effort to find a physician who is skilled at the procedure.

If the fibroid is growing into the uterine cavity (submucous), the doctor can schedule outpatient surgery called resectoscopic myomectomy, notes Steven R. Goldstein, M.D., professor of obstetrics and gynecology at New York University School of Medicine in New York City and director of gynecologic ultrasound at the university's medical center. "If the doctor has the equipment and the know-how, this isn't much more involved than a D and C." From the patient's point of view, there is no incision, and there's little recovery time.

The myomectomy becomes more complicated if the fibroid is on the outside wall of the uterus (subserous) or within the muscular wall (intramural). Even so, the myomectomy can be done by using a laparoscope on an outpatient basis under general anesthesia, and pain and recovery time are minimal.

The more complex myomectomies are done with a larger abdominal incision under general anesthesia. The uterus is opened, the fibroids are removed, and the uterus is then reconstructed. These are most often done on women who have the most fibroids, large fibroids, or fibroids in difficult locations, or on women who plan to have children. Howard A. Zacur, M.D., Ph.D., professor of reproductive endocrinology and director of the estrogen consultation service at Johns Hopkins Medical Institutions in Baltimore, notes, "It entails a recovery comparable to any other major abdominal surgery." Still, abdominal myomectomy may be easier for women than abdominal hysterectomy.

There's one big drawback to all myomectomies: Fibroids grow back in about 15 to 30 percent of women who've had one. These women may need repeat procedures—or even, eventually, hysterectomies.

Alternative medicine is not reported to be very helpful for shrinking fibroids, but it has helped some women control some of the symptoms.

Abnormal Bleeding

What is it? Heavy or abnormal bleeding, also called dysfunctional uterine bleeding, leads to a fifth of all hysterectomies in the United States.

What are the symptoms? To some women, it means very heavy periods. Others have unpredictable bleeding throughout their cycles. In severe cases, it can lead to anemia. And sometimes, it is a sign of precancerous or cancerous conditions.

How is it best diagnosed? Abnormal bleeding calls for a thorough investigation, and that should start with a detailed history. The most important question is: Is the bleeding cyclical, or is it unpredictable?

For women with irregular bleeding throughout their cycles, a Pap

Weighing the Decision

Hysterectomy is risky, it's complicated, and it's not a sure thing. What's more, some of the medical literature says that as many as 50 percent of women who have had them report new problems after the surgery, including urinary incontinence, pelvic pain, loss of sexual desire, reduction in orgasm, premature menopause (even when the ovaries are left in place), and depression.

But, on the other hand, for women who are incapacitated by fibroids, for example, hysterectomies can really be freeing. In fact, a well-done recent study from Harvard Medical School followed 418 women for a year after they had hysterectomies and found that there was a significant improvement in their quality of life, while few women found they had new problems.

And, of course, hysterectomy is warranted—indeed, absolutely necessary—under certain circumstances, notably, for invasive cancer of the uterus. "There really isn't a safe alternative to hysterectomy," says Brian Walsh, M.D., director of the Menopause Clinic at Brigham and Women's Hospital in Boston. For most cases of invasive cancer of the cervix and ovaries, hysterectomies are usually needed, too. That's because those cancers usually spread through the uterus. The exception is if you have very early cervical cancer and are determined to keep your uterus. The option then is extensive cone biopsy—removal of the affected areas. Talk to your physician about it.

Dr. Walsh points out that invasive cancer is different from precancers of the cervix and uterus. Precancers of the cervix can be treated with local surgery, and uterine precancers can be treated with hormones. "Often, hormones work, but if not, a hysterectomy might be needed later."

Keep in mind, however, that cancer doesn't account for the vast majority of hysterectomies. Dr. Walsh estimates that, in all, cancer accounts for fewer than five percent.

So what do you do when your doctor recommends hysterectomy? First, check out all of your options thoroughly. Then, Dr. Walsh counsels his patients to look inside themselves for the answers. "Most of my patients know what they want," he adds, "but some come in and say 'Do I go for myomectomy or hysterectomy?' I say, 'Intuitively, deep down inside, what feels right for you?' A patient might say, 'I know that childbearing is not an issue for me, but I really want my uterus; it's part of me.' I say, 'Then you should keep it.'"

"I Said No to Hysterectomy"

Nancy, 46, is a fund-raising executive for a nonprofit organization in upstate New York.

"About a year ago, my periods started getting longer and heavier, to the point where they lasted two weeks, and I was changing pads constantly. Meetings and airplane rides meant constant stress—would I bleed through my clothes? It was almost impossible to maintain my daily routine.

"At first, I assumed I was just approaching menopause. But then I figured I better have it checked out.

"My doctor examined me. Her diagnosis was a single large fibroid tumor in the uterus. She told me to start thinking about a hysterectomy.

"My immediate gut reaction was, 'I don't want a hysterectomy!' She said, 'Do you plan to have more children?' I said no, and she chuckled. She dismissed me with a prescription for birth control pills and told me to come back in six months if they didn't work.

"The next day, I went to the library. I live in a small town, but the library had a stack of books with titles like *You Don't Need a Hysterectomy*. I took out five of them. The next day, my fiancé and I were driving to Philadelphia, and while he drove, I read out loud. By the time we arrived, we were both adamantly opposed to hysterectomy, and we knew there were alternatives.

"One book gave the name of the HERS (Hysterectomy Educational Resources and Services) Foundation (an organization in Bala Cynwyd, Pennsylvania, that counsels women about hysterectomy). I made an appointment to talk to the director, Nora Coffey. Based on my symptoms, she told me the type of fibroid I probably had was a pedunculated fibroid, which means that it's growing on a stalk. She told me that this

smear and endometrial sampling—to look for precancerous or cancerous cells in the cervix or uterus—is vital. This means scraping some cells from the cervix or uterus. "I do it in the office, and it takes about 10 seconds and causes a little cramping," says Dr. Walsh. It's also important to do an ultrasound to locate possible growths, such as fibroids, that are causing the bleeding. For women with regular but heavy periods, biopsy is not as vital, but an ultrasound can supply important diagnostic information.

When is a hysterectomy inappropriate? Hysterectomies are not ap-

was one of the easiest fibroids to remove and to ask for a shelling out of the fibroid, called resectoscopic surgery.

"She gave me the names of several doctors in Boston, New York City, and Philadelphia, but I decided to try to find a doctor in my area who could perform the procedure. I called the top teaching hospital here and made an appointment with the doctor who was said to know how to do the resectoscopy. The first thing he said was, 'Tell me why you don't want a hysterectomy.' When I told him about some of the problems that I had read about, he dismissed each one of them. He said, 'Many women report that they never felt better than after hysterectomies.' Then he went on to say that I was a prime candidate for resectoscopic surgery, but he would still need permission to do a hysterectomy if necessary. I refused. He told me to go find another doctor.

"I made another appointment with Nora Coffey. 'Stop messing around with those doctors. Go to one that I told you about,' she said. So I called the doctor in Boston. When I got to his office, I raised the question of hysterectomy. He looked me right in the eye and said, 'I have done hundreds of fibroid removals, and I have never had to do a hysterectomy.'

"So last November, my fiancé and I drove to Boston. The surgery (a vaginal, not abdominal, procedure) lasted two hours under full anesthesia. I woke up a little nauseated from the anesthesia, but I was back at the motel by 9:00 P.M., and was in the car, on the way home, by 10:00 A.M. the next day. One day later, I went to work.

"I can't tell you how hard it is when you're having the kind of bleeding that I was experiencing, and someone is offering you a hysterectomy as an out, how tempting it is to take them up on it.

"It was hard to keep looking for answers. But I'm glad I did."

propriate when the cause of the bleeding hasn't been diagnosed or when medications such as hormones haven't yet been tried. Most experts agree that hysterectomy should only be considered as a last resort. According to some experts, fewer than 10 percent of cases of genuine abnormal bleeding should require hysterectomies.

What are the alternatives? Depending on the cause of the bleeding, treatments might include the following:

NSAIDs can sometimes help slow down bleeding.

Combination oral contraceptives (OCs) are often ideal for women who are not ovulating regularly and are therefore bleeding throughout the month. "OCs can give wonderful regularity," says Dr. Walsh. And they can help ward off the risk of endometrial cancer, a disease which is more likely to strike women with irregular ovulation.

Progesterone can be helpful for women with irregular ovulation leading to unusual bleeding. Dr. Walsh often uses it for women who don't want to take or can't tolerate birth control pills.

How does it work? Progesterone is the hormone that makes the lining of the uterus grow, and when it withdraws, the lining sheds. "If you don't have progesterone," Dr. Walsh explains, "this lining gets thicker until it gets very unstable, and a little piece may fall off, and sometimes you have spotting. Other times a whole chunk falls off, and you have very heavy bleeding." Taking a progestin for 10 to 14 days can regularize the cycle. (For women who cannot tolerate synthetic progestins, natural progesterone can be a more comfortable choice.)

Endometrial ablation is another alternative to hysterectomy. In this procedure, the endometrium (the inner lining of the uterus) and the basilis (the layer under it) are destroyed. "We can do it vaginally. It's a minor procedure, and you can keep your uterus," says Dr. Fugh-Berman. "It's permanent, but it's much less invasive than hysterectomy."

The success rates of endometrial ablation are good. Studies show fewer complications and much shorter hospital stays and recovery periods compared with hysterectomy.

Perhaps the number one drawback is that ablation is not as complete a solution for bleeding as hysterectomy is. "No matter which technique is used, a third of patients will have no more bleeding," says Dr. Walsh. "A third will have spotting or a light flow that needs a panty liner. Twenty-five percent will have average periods. And about 5 to 10 percent are no better afterward than they were before." Another downside is that ablation leaves the woman infertile.

After menopause, women who have had ablations and wish to take estrogen replacement therapy will need a progestin, too. That's because ablation might disguise one of the key symptoms of endometrial cancer—bleeding.

Because of the downsides, says Dr. Goldstein, many of his patients use medication to keep bleeding to a minimum and opt for neither ablation nor hysterectomy. Once they're through menopause, then bleeding won't be an issue any more, provided they're not taking HRT.

Endometriosis

What is it? In endometriosis, bits of the lining of the uterus grow outside the uterus in the abdomen and on the ovaries. Fueled by estrogen, the tissue then grows and bleeds on a monthly cycle. This can lead to chronic pain, inflammation, scar tissue, and other problems. After menopause, endometriosis tends to go away, unless a woman takes HRT.

The causes of endometriosis are unknown, but theories include a genetic tendency, stray endometrial cells that may flow back through the fallopian tubes and settle in the pelvis, exposure to toxins, and there's even the possibility that it is an autoimmune disorder. Endometriosis causes about a fifth of all hysterectomies in the United States.

What are the symptoms? Endometriosis is linked to chronic pelvic pain—especially during menstruation, intercourse, and urination—and also to infertility and other problems.

How is it best diagnosed? The diagnosis is made with a laparoscopy, an outpatient procedure done under general anesthesia. The doctor inserts a slender optical instrument through a small incision in the lower abdomen to look around for growths of endometrial tissue. "We're still looking for effective noninvasive ways to diagnose endometriosis, but they're not here yet," says Tess Thompson, support program coordinator for the Endometriosis Association, an international self-help organization based in Milwaukee.

When is a hysterectomy inappropriate? A hysterectomy alone may not be considered an effective treatment for endometriosis. Frequently, the ovaries have to be removed, too, to help stop the endometrial tissue implants from growing. And even then, it doesn't always work. "For some women with severe, advanced endometriosis with well-documented scar tissue, sometimes a hysterectomy and oophorectomy (removal of the ovaries) have to be resorted to, but that's in a very small number of people," says Dr. Goldstein.

What are the alternatives? Endometriosis can't be cured. But it can be controlled. Here's how.

NSAIDs can be used for pain. A woman who doesn't respond to one type might respond to another.

Oral contraceptives alter the balance of estrogen and progesterone, slowing the progression of endometriosis, says Dr. Walsh. OCs are most effective for milder cases, he adds.

GnRH agonists are powerful hormones that block estrogen and shrink endometrial tissue. The most commonly used ones for endometriosis are Synarel and Lupron. One problem, though, is that they have powerful side effects, especially Lupron. "It's like menopause with a vengeance," says Dr. Walsh. These drugs are usually not a long-term solution. Women don't use them for more than a few months, mainly because they could lose bone from estrogen deprivation, but they might get a woman to pregnancy or to the point where OCs can maintain her progress, or they might make surgery easier.

Outpatient laparoscopic surgery can be performed during the same procedure in which endometriosis is diagnosed. The stray endometrial growths can be destroyed with an electrical device or a laser. The disease does have a tendency to recur, but birth control pills can help maintain the regression.

A laparotomy may be required for more extensive disease, entailing more and larger abdominal incisions, a few days in the hospital, and longer recovery time.

Alternative medicine has provided some women with good results, especially when conventional medicine is combined with approaches like Traditional Chinese Medicine, herbs, nutrition, supplements, and other alternative treatments.

Sage Advice

Take Steps to Block Breast Cancer

Does exercising reduce your chances of getting breast cancer? One of the biggest investigations ever done on the topic suggests that the answer is yes. Researchers in Norway traced the health of more than 25,000 women over a nine-year period. They found that women who exercised at least four hours a week had a 37 percent lower breast cancer risk compared with women who did no exercise at all. They also found that women who were very active at work—those whose jobs involved lots of lifting and walking—reduced risk by about a fourth.

Does this mean that you should run out and get a job delivering pianos? That would be premature (and a bad career move). But taking the stairs instead of the elevator, using the copier down the hall, and otherwise being more active in your day-to-day life could help. "We're not sure how much exercise women need to do," says Anne McTiernan, M.D., Ph.D., of the Fred Hutchinson Cancer Research Center in Seattle. "But we do know that women who are overweight have an increased risk of breast cancer."

Of course, says Dr. McTiernan, "the more exercise you do, the better." That's true for a host of reasons, ranging from lower blood pressure to reduced risk of diabetes. Breast cancer risk hasn't been definitively added to that list . . . yet. But exercise now, and odds are, you won't regret it later.

Reducing Your Risk with a Few Rays a Day

Sunshine brings an unexpected health benefit to women at risk for breast cancer. Researchers who studied health data on nearly 5,000 women found that breast cancer risk in women who reported getting the most sun exposure was about 30 to 40 percent lower than the risk among women who got the least sun. A similar reduction in risk was found among women who lived in sunny climes.

The key to this phenomenon may be vitamin D, which is produced in our skin when it's exposed to sunlight. It only takes about 10 to 15 minutes of sun exposure a day to get the vitamin D that your body needs, says the study's author, Esther John, Ph.D., an epidemiologist at the Northern California Cancer Center in Union City. "And that's just casual exposure—the sunlight you get on your face and neck and arms and hands when you're regularly dressed," she explains. So while the exact dose of sunlight needed is unknown, taking a brief outdoor stroll (without sunscreen) seems a prudent way to try to benefit from the sun's cancer-fighting power. (Prolonged, unprotected exposure to sunlight should be avoided since it raises your risk of skin cancer.)

Getting vitamin D in your diet (primarily from milk) and from supplements may also help, says Dr. John, epecially if you live in northern latitudes, where a multivitamin with 400 international units (IU), the Daily Value, may be beneficial. (But don't try for too much vitamin D. Levels well above 600 IU on a regular basis can be harmful.)

A Warning for Working Women

If your job is stressing you out, more than your mind is being frazzled: Your health may be in jeopardy as well. In a study of 152 women, those who reported high levels of job strain also scored high for depression, anxiety, neuroticism, and hostility—factors that leave them more vulnerable.

How do you know if you're at risk? According to the study's director, *Prevention* advisor Redford B. Williams, M.D., professor of psychiatry and director of the Behavioral Medicine Research Center at Duke University School of Medicine in Durham, North Carolina, women suffering from job strain were more socially isolated.

"Being more irritable with family, finding that you're not really interacting very much with friends, not attending religious activities as much—all these would be signals that your job and your psyche are interacting in ways that are potentially dangerous to your health." The solution? "I would suggest aerobic exercise. Vigorous exercise is very helpful in washing out the badness, clearing away the negative cobwebs." Another antidote is talking about your problems with friends. "Telling what you experienced, rather than making a value judgment like 'my boss is a jerk,' is an effective way to get a friend to be sympathetic."

Help Yourself to a More Comfortable Mammogram

Getting a mammogram doesn't have to be an unpleasant experience, says John Coscia, M.D., director of clinical breast radiology at the

University of Texas Southwestern Medical Center at Dallas. Not every woman finds the procedure uncomfortable, but if you do, his suggestions should make things easier.

- Schedule your exam during the time in your menstrual cycle when your breasts are the least tender. For most women, this is in the first two weeks of the cycle. (According to one study, having a mammogram during this time may also improve accuracy for women of childbearing age.)
- Cut off caffeine, especially coffee, for a week before the exam. "There's good anecdotal evidence that this can help," says Dr. Coscia, though the reason why isn't clear. Taking vitamin E for a few weeks beforehand (400 to 800 international units, or IUs, a day) also seems to help.
- Take an over-the-counter pain reliever about an hour beforehand. Use it afterward, too, if needed.
- Speak up if you're feeling uncomfortable during the procedure. "The patient should be in control of the exam," says Dr. Coscia. "The breast is compressed against the x-ray plate to improve accuracy, but there's room for adjustment." The technologist giving the exam should be able to make you comfortable without sacrificing the effectiveness of the mammogram.

What to Eat with the Pill

If you take an oral contraceptive, you may want to add more carrots, yams, or broccoli to your diet. In a study of 610 women, researchers in Germany found that among women over age 24, beta-carotene levels tended to be lower in oral contraceptive users compared with nonusers. This effect was particularly strong in women ages 35 to 44. In these women, oral contraceptive use had a stronger impact on beta-carotene levels than smoking is known to have. Other studies show that people whose diets are high in beta-carotene have lower risks of heart disease and cancer.

According to Nancy Potischman, Ph.D., a nutritional epidemiologist with the National Cancer Institute, the oral contraceptive study is "provocative, though not conclusive." While researchers examine this study further, it's smart to stock up on fruits and vegetables that are high in beta-carotene. Yellow and orange vegetables are your best bet.

Cancer Protection in a Bean

Do soybeans help sideline cancer? One clue is that in Asia, where women get regular helpings of soy foods, the risk of breast cancer is lower than in America.

Now we have another indication that soy protects breasts. In a study of almost 1,600 Asian-American women in California and Hawaii, those eating tofu (soybean curd) once a week had almost one-third less chance of getting breast cancer compared with those eating tofu only once a month.

And the amazing soybean may ward off another serious illness that strikes nearly 35,000 American women a year: endometrial cancer. A Hawaiian study found that women who regularly eat the most soy products such as tofu, soy milk, and roasted soy nuts have less than half the risk of endometrial cancer compared with women who eat no soy. We need more proof, but it's interesting that rates of endometrial cancer are lower in Asia, where most women eat soy every day.

Never Too Late to Boost Bone

When you skipped hormone replacement therapy (HRT) at menopause, you and your doctor deemed it best. But it's a decade later, your tennis partner is wearing a cast instead of wristbands, and you're wondering if bypassing estrogen (and its now well-documented bone benefit) could put you on the sidelines.

Good news: Research suggests that later-in-life estrogen therapy can boost bone protection for many women, even if begun 10 to 15 years after menopause. In fact, within 9 years, women who had started the hormone after the age of 60 had nearly identical bone densities as those having taken it for 20 years since menopause.

Bone health is just one factor in the decision to begin, or continue, estrogen replacement therapy, notes study co-author Elizabeth L. Barrett-Connor, M.D., professor at the University of California, San Diego. Others include menopausal symptoms and family history of heart disease or breast cancer. It is concern about estrogen's association with the latter that has made some physicians reluctant to prescribe it for long-term use.

"But health risks shift over time, and threats of hip fracture and heart disease catch up to and exceed any cancer risk for many women as they enter their seventies," says Dr. Barrett-Connor. "For that reason, belated estrogen may be a strong option for those who find osteoporosis now near the top of their priorities list." (Short-term estrogen replacement—for five years following menopause, for example—may ease other symptoms, but appears to offer no long-term protection from brittle bones.)

Exercise with Confidence

Running and other high-impact activities do not contribute to long-term urinary incontinence problems, according to a recent study. Researchers checked with 104 former Olympic athletes, now over age 40, to find out if those who participated in high-impact events such as gymnastics and track and field had more problems with urinary leakage than low-impact swimmers.

The high-impact athletes were no more likely to have incontinence problems than the swimmers were. Although these findings need to be confirmed, most of us aren't training at the intensity of Olympic athletes, so the likelihood of our developing urinary incontinence due to exercise is probably even less.

Nevertheless, the leakage of urine during exercise is common among women. So, if you have this problem, here are some home remedies.
- Empty your bladder frequently.
- Get a good night's sleep. Fatigued pelvic muscles have trouble holding your bladder closed.
- Try cutting back on spicy and tomato-based foods, alcohol, coffee, chocolate, citrus, and other acidic foods. They can increase the need to urinate.
- Strengthen pelvic muscles. Kegel exercises (tightening the pelvic muscles as if to stop urinating), can help restore bladder control.

The Citrus Cancer Chaser

Every glass of citrus juice you drink may strike a blow against breast cancer, suggests a study at the University of Western Ontario in Canada.

Researchers gave mice either double-strength orange or grapefruit juice or plain drinking water. After the mice were injected with human breast cancer cells, the juice groups got 50 percent fewer tumors, and the tumors were 50 percent less likely to spread. What did it? Two special compounds, hesperidin in oranges and naringin in grapefruit, may be partly responsible, researchers say. Keep in mind that what works in animals doesn't always work in people. More studies are needed find that out. And no one is suggesting that you drink nothing but juice. But doesn't a nice cold glass of orange juice sound sweeter than ever?

Herbal Elixirs

Mother Nature's Coolest, Smartest Menopause Remedies

The variety can make you dizzy, whether you're in menopause or not. There's Born Again cream, Menopause Support capsules, Easy Change gel, and Women's Balance tablets, to name a few. Visit any health food supermarket, and you're likely to find more than 40 different potions in the change-of-life section.

And the prices may even give your husband a hot flash: A three-week supply of cream runs a cool $24.99. Sixty vitamin supplements costs $15.99. A delicate two-ounce vial of herbal tincture carries a $12.99 price tag.

Do these products actually do what their names imply? Will they take away the hot flashes, vaginal dryness, night sweats, mood swings, or other symptoms that can make menopause seem like such a hassle?

According to some experts, some of the promises are true—but only some. Leaders in the fields of menopause and natural therapies say that there are sound reasons to believe that a number of health food store products might safely alleviate some discomforts of menopause. And there are sound reasons to believe that others won't.

Since so many combination products are on the shelves but so few have been tested, it's smartest to look at these remedies in terms of individual ingredients. Here's what's what.

Tips for Smart Consumers

When you go the health food store route for menopause, keep these points in mind.

- Store clerks are not medical authorities. "Some have very good intentions," says Gail Mahady, R.Ph., Ph.D., research assistant professor at the University of Illinois College of Pharmacy, Chicago, program for collaborative research in the pharmaceutical sciences, "but they don't have adequate scientific backgrounds to counsel people."
- Be wary of ultra-combination products. Herbs and nutrients often come in mixtures. For example, some menopause products contain black cohosh, ginseng, chasteberry, and sometimes zillions of other things, too.

  "You can only stuff so much into one capsule," says Tori Hudson, N.D., a naturopathic physician and professor at the National College of Naturopathic Medicine in Portland, Oregon. "If there are more than six ingredients, there's probably a very small amount of each, so the therapeutic benefit of any one herb goes down."
- Be wary of creams. Whether the labels boast of black cohosh, chasteberry, wild yam, or some of the other medicinal herbs, they may not be absorbed sufficiently through the skin to be active.
- If you do try an herbal or nutrient product, give it time to work. Dr. Mahady suggests up to about three months. "After that, if you don't see an improvement, try something different."
- Take the right dose. Don't use less, or more. "Part of the reason that herbs don't seem to work is that people tend not to take

Compared with Estrogen . . .

How does the health food store route compare with hormone replacement therapy? Here are a few important ways.

Pluses

• Some prescription estrogens are plant-derived, while some, most notably, Premarin, contain estrogen extracted from pregnant mares' urine. For women who want to avoid those forms of prescription estrogen that do come from animals, the herbal remedies may be a good option.

• Experts are optimistic that some of the herbs used for menopause don't cause endometrial cancer or possibly increase the risk of breast cancer, unlike estrogen. For example, European studies have not shown that black cohosh promotes breast cancer or other estrogen-related cancers. However, no one has studied the long-term effects of any of the other herbs on cancer.

Minuses

• Unlike estrogen, no single herb is proven to prevent osteoporosis.

• The alternative products may work best for mild symptoms. If a woman has very severe symptoms, she might respond much better to conventional hormone replacement therapy.

• Alternative products can be just as expensive as prescription products.

things in the recommended dose—they think they're going to save money," says Dr. Hudson. On the other side of the spectrum, overdoing it can cause harmful side effects.

• Women who are pregnant or lactating shouldn't use herbs without a medical consultation.

• Don't take any herbal products if you're on birth control pills or on hormone replacement therapy without consulting your doctor. She may need to adjust your dose if the herbs contain plant hormones.

• Buy from a company whose name you know and whose other products you may already trust. "The amounts of herbs or nutrients in the jars are probably not dangerous as long as they contain what they say they do," says herb expert and *Prevention* advisor Varro E. Tyler, Ph.D., Sc.D. "But there have been cases where disreputable companies adulterated their products, and people were hurt as a result."

Herbal Inventory

Black cohosh (*Cimicifuga racemosa*): often helpful

What it does: Evidence suggests that it can relieve hot flashes, night sweats, headaches, heart palpitations, and vaginal drying and thinning. The best documented of all the herbal remedies, black cohosh has been shown to suppress the secretion of luteinizing hormone (LH), a hormone that's believed to be at the root of many of these symptoms. Some studies suggest that black cohosh can reduce menopause-related headaches, depression, anxiety, and decreased libido, points out Dr. Tyler.

How we know: European studies confirm that black cohosh relieves many menopausal symptoms. In fact, one double-blind study of 80 women found that it reduced menopausal symptoms better than the conjugated estrogens did. Black cohosh has been approved for the treatment of menopausal symptoms by Commission E, Germany's leading authority entrusted with evaluating the safety and efficacy of herb remedies.

Products available: Capsules, tablets, drops, powders. (Capsules or drops are the most practical way to take black cohosh; the dose is too small to take as a tea.)

Note: There are many brands of black cohosh. But there's one brand in particular that many experts say they trust: Remifemin. The brand has been around for decades in Europe, and it became available in the United States in 1996. Its quality and dose are controlled by a reputable manufacturer, and many of the European studies were done with Remifemin.

How much to take: Forty milligrams a day is the therapeutic dose approved by Commission E. Many products contain more—sometimes hundreds of milligrams more—but larger doses are unnecessary and may even be unsafe. Be sure to read the label to know how much of a product you need to take to get the equivalent of 40 milligrams of black cohosh.

Cautions: Black cohosh can require time and money. "It takes at least three to four weeks before the effects kick in. Some women want relief tomorrow, or yesterday," notes menopause expert Dixie Mills, M.D., clinical assistant professor of surgery at the University of Vermont in Burlington.

Black cohosh therapy can also be more expensive than prescription estrogen. Premarin (the most widely dispensed brand of estrogen) costs less than 40 cents a day, while Remifemin (at the recommended dose of two 20-milligram tablets daily) runs about 50 to 60 cents a day. Unlike estrogen replacement therapy, black cohosh isn't able to help prevent osteoporosis or possibly prevent cardiovascular disease.

Dr. Tyler notes that some people report upset stomachs from black cohosh. Because the long-term toxicity has not been studied, he agrees with the Commission E recommendation that women use it for no longer than six months continuously. Dr. Tyler suggests allowing several weeks between uses.

Chasteberry (*Vitex agnus-castus*): possibly helpful

What it might do: Relieve hot flashes, night sweats, headaches, heart palpitations, and vaginal drying and thinning. Even though Commission E has approved chasteberry for treating symptoms of menopause, Dr. Tyler has a hunch that it's not so helpful for this time of life. Based on the herb's pharmacology, it is believed to reduce levels of prolactin, a hormone associated with PMS symptoms. "There's much more research showing that it is effective for premenstrual syndrome, and that makes more sense to me," says Dr. Tyler.

How we know: Germany's Commission E has approved chasteberry for treating symptoms of menopause. In clinical experience, experts' reviews of its effectiveness have been mixed.

Products available: Pills, tea, drops; alone and in various combinations.

How much to take: The therapeutic dose for menopause recommended by Commission E is 20 milligrams a day. "Capsules or drops are a practical way to take chasteberry," says Dr. Tyler. "But if you wish, you can make a tea. Use a pinch of powdered chasteberry (approximately 20 milligrams), and steep it in hot water for 15 minutes. Drink a cup once a day."

Cautions: While the side effects and long-term toxicity aren't well-documented, we do know that chasteberry can trigger rashes in some people. It should not be used by women experiencing reduced sexual desire as part of their menopause: The herbal literature reports that it reduces libido. (Another name for this herb is monk's pepper, and it really was used in monasteries.)

Ginseng (*Panax ginseng*): possibly helpful

What it might do: Erase some of the fatigue and possibly even slight depression that can come with menopause. Ginseng is a proven stimulant, notes Dr. Tyler, and in menopause, it may give a boost to your general feelings of well-being.

Some doctors believe that it might have an estrogen-like effect on the body, easing menopausal symptoms, such as vaginal dryness and hot flashes, and possibly stimulating endometrial growth and bleeding. Some women who take ginseng experience uterine bleeding long after they have gone through menopause, says Brian Walsh, M.D., director of the menopause clinic at Brigham and Women's Hospital in Boston. With such a lack of research, the unanswered question is whether bleeding can be attributed to the herb itself or to the use of an inferior product.

How we know: Its effect as a stimulant is beginning to be documented in rigorous scientific studies. Two recent investigations involving more than 500 people suggest that people taking ginseng—combined with vitamins and minerals—felt an improved quality of life. Other studies suggest boosts in psychological well-being and energy. But the evidence of an effect on specific menopause symptoms is at this point only anecdotal.

Products available: Capsules, drops, tea bags, dried herb; alone and in combination.

How much to take: No one knows the therapeutic dose for menopause, since this remedy is unproven. But for other uses, the recommended dose of a typical product containing 4 percent ginsenosides is two 100-milligram capsules daily. Capsules or drops are a practical way to take ginseng. Or you can make a tea. Steep one teaspoonful of the dried product for about 10 to 15 minutes, once a day, Dr. Tyler suggests.

If ginseng is already in your menopause remedy but the label doesn't say how much of the active ingredient is in there, Dr. Tyler has this advice: If you find that you can't sleep at night, you're probably taking too much.

If any type of ginseng could be effective for menopause, it would be *Panax ginseng.* This is the variety on which most studies have been done. Other forms of ginseng, such as *Panax quinquefolius,* have not been as well-studied.

Cautions: None.

Vitamin E (not an herb, but worth mentioning): possibly helpful

What it might do: Decrease hot flashes.

How we know: Anecdotal evidence and clinical experience. Dr. Walsh says that many of his patients have reported that vitamin E seems to reduce their hot flashes. "It makes sense," he says, "when you consider that vitamin E is structurally similar to estrogen at the molecular level." So it might act as a mild form of estrogen replacement therapy, he explains.

Unfortunately, there are no well-controlled, large-scale studies that prove vitamin E reduces menopause symptoms. But many women and doctors, based on their experience, feel that it helps. In a survey of *Prevention* magazine readers' menopause remedies, conducted in 1992, half of the women who tried vitamin E for hot flashes and night sweats reported improvements in their symptoms.

Products available: Pills, in combination products, and alone.

How much to take: Experts suggest 40 to 800 international units (IU) daily.

Caution: If you are considering taking amounts of vitamin E above 200 IU, discuss this with your doctor first. A study using low-dose vitamin E supplements showed an increased risk of hemorrhagic stroke.

Licorice root (*Glycyrrhiza glabra*): approach cautiously

What it might do: Reduce hot flashes, irregular bleeding, mood swings, and vaginal dryness. Licorice root contains high levels of estrogen-like compounds, called phytoestrogens, that act like a weak estrogen in some parts of the body. That means phytoestrogens might have the ability to act like hormone replacement therapy, quashing hot flashes and other symptoms that are believed to result from the reduction in estrogen levels that comes with menopause. However, unlike soy, another food high in phytoestrogens, licorice root has the potential for side effects and can't be recommended, as soy can be.

How we know: Anecdotal evidence and speculation. "There are simply no studies that show licorice root can affect symptoms of menopause in human beings," says Dr. Tyler. While this is similar to what is known for remedies like vitamin E, licorice root is in the "approach cautiously" category because of its potential for sometimes serious side effects.

Soy Soldiers to the Rescue

While a multitude of herbs are touted for helping menopause symptoms, a better aid might be the lowly soybean.

"Tofu and other soy products may be more promising for menopause than any herbs," says herb expert and *Prevention* advisor Varro E. Tyler, Ph.D., Sc.D. Soy may be effective for soothing hot flashes, eliminating vaginal dryness, slowing bone loss, and protecting the heart. No one can say for sure how much you need, but many experts think that taking in soy products containing 30 to 50 milligrams of isoflavones a day may be enough. That's about 1½ cups of low-fat soy milk, ½ cup of tofu, or 2 tablespoons of roasted soy nuts.

Products available: Pills, drops, tea bags, and in bulk; alone and in combination.

How much to take: If you're still determined to try this, and you have your doctor's okay, at least use a safe dose. According to Germany's Commission E, that's up to 15 grams a day, for no longer than four weeks. To get 15 grams from tea, you'd need to steep two to three teaspoons of the dried product for 10 to 15 minutes and drink three to four cups a day. If taking it in other forms, check the label for the right amount to equal 15 grams.

Cautions: Licorice root really shouldn't be used without consulting a doctor. Licorice contains compounds that affect the adrenal hormones in potentially harmful ways. "It can raise blood pressure and lower potassium, and there's even a reported case of a cardiac arrest," says Adriane Fugh-Berman, M.D., chairwoman of the National Women's Health Network, an independent consumer advocacy organization in Washington, D.C.; nationally recognized authority on alternative medicine; and author of *Alternative Medicine: What Works.* While the trouble in these cases was caused by people addicted to licorice laxatives or imported licorice candy (black licorice in this country is flavored with anise, not real licorice), "that doesn't negate the fact that high doses of licorice can be harmful," she adds. The point is, it shouldn't be used without consulting a doctor or other health care practitioner knowledgeable about herbs.

Dong quai; also spelled dong kwai (*Angelica sinensis*): probably not helpful

What it probably won't do: Relieve any symptoms of menopause. The best that dong quai can offer are compounds in it that make it a mild laxative and central nervous system stimulant.

How we know: There has been at least one well-controlled clinical study on dong quai for menopausal women in the United States, and it showed no benefit.

"If anything, dong quai lowers the circulating levels of estradiol (one of the body's own estrogens), rather than raising them," says David T. Zava, Ph.D., who has researched this herb and who is one of the nation's leading experts on plant estrogens. Dr. Zava is the director of the Aeron LifeCycle hormone testing laboratory in San Leandro, California.

One reason why some reports may have turned up positive for anti-menopause effects is that in Traditional Chinese Medicine—where this herb and menopause have been linked—dong quai is always combined with other herbs. Dr. Zava speculates that this herb may need to be complemented with other herbs to be helpful.

Products available: Pills, drops, powder in bulk; alone and in various combinations.

Cautions: Dong quai can cause skin problems, especially when skin is exposed to the sun. "Women who use it should wear sunscreen," says Dr. Tyler.

Gail Mahady, R.Ph., Ph.D., research assistant professor at the University of Illinois College of Pharmacy, Chicago, program for collaborative research in the pharmaceutical sciences, adds another important caution: "Dong quai is not for women who have excessive vaginal bleeding; it might make it worse."

Label Decoder

In addition to the herbs listed above, you'll probably see many others that make numerous claims. On those many shelves of menopause remedies, for example, you see progesterone products bearing the words "wild yam extract," "diosgenin," and of course, "natural" on the labels. Intriguing labels, but what do they signify? What these progesterone products can and can't do for menopause is a subject of hot debate, and the scientific jury is still out on their usefulness.

In the meantime, you should at least know what you're getting or not getting if your practitioner has recommended that you try them.

• A product contains natural progesterone if the progesterone is biologically identical to what your body makes. The term *natural* doesn't refer to the source of the progesterone.

• Wild yams contain a compound called diosgenin, which can be converted to progesterone like your body makes, but it can only be done in a lab. This conversion must take place before it is added to a product, since diosgenin can't be converted to progesterone by the body. If the label says, for example, 10 percent diosgenin, you're not getting progesterone, only the extract of the wild yam that was never chemically made into progesterone.

• If you see "progesterone (USP)" on the label, it means that the manufacturer has added pharmaceutical-grade natural progesterone (derived from diosgenin) to the mix. Products containing about 400 to 1,000 milligrams (1.5 to 3 percent) of progesterone per ounce are likely to be the most clinically effective, according to Dr. Zava.

• More manufacturers of over-the-counter progesterone products are listing the amounts of progesterone that they contain. However, some labels can be vague or confusing. Don't hesitate to contact manufacturers to ask what amounts of progesterone their products contain, especially if you don't even see progesterone listed on the labels.

Don't Forget the Big Picture

No matter which herbs you choose or reject for menopause symptoms, it's essential to keep the big picture in mind. Treating individual menopause symptoms with herbs may bring relief now, but it could mean neglecting the two most significant life-threatening problems related to menopause: osteoporosis and cardiovascular disease, according to Tori Hudson, N.D., a naturopathic physician and professor at the National College of Naturopathic Medicine in Portland, Oregon. As a naturopath, Dr. Hudson has trained at an accredited four-year naturopathic medical school. Naturopaths manage menopause by aiming to avoid drugs, but Dr. Hudson does refer people to prescription estrogens if she feels that such treatment is needed.

Absolute musts for all menopausal women are risk assessments for both osteoporosis and cardiovascular disease. More important, a complete evaluation can help you and your doctor sort out whether you might be helped by some of the herbal and vitamin-based health food store products or whether you need hormone therapy with estrogen or progesterone.

The bottom line is that decisions about menopause treatments, especially natural menopause treatments, should be made with the help of a knowledgeable medical professional who is aware of all the options—herbs as well as different hormone therapies.

There's no question: The products in the health food store can increase your options during menopause. But it's vital to do your homework first.

"I think people have to realize that natural pharmacy companies, just like conventional pharmaceutical companies, are very hip to the demographics of menopause," says Dr. Hudson. "It's a big business, and with more women coming into menopause, everybody wants a piece of the action." So stick with what's been shown to be most effective and safe, what makes you feel good, and what's right for you.

Home Remedies

Block Yeast Infections with Beta-Carotene

Crunch on carrots to prevent yeast infections? Not a bad idea. According to doctors in the department of obstetrics and gynecology at Albert Einstein College of Medicine of Yeshiva University in New York City, eating carrots and other foods rich in beta-carotene—a natural substance that's converted into vitamin A in the body—may offer some protection against yeast infections. In one study, vaginal cells in women with yeast infections had significantly lower levels of beta-carotene than did the vaginal cells in women who did not have yeast infections. The doctors theorize that this benefit may be due to beta-carotene's ability to boost the immune system.

Spinach, broccoli, sweet potatoes, and apricots, in addition to carrots, all contain plentiful amounts of beta-carotene.

To Eat or Not to Eat for Nausea

Whether you're suffering from morning sickness or motion sickness, or you're just plain nauseated for no good reason, the fact is, you feel rotten. And the last thing you want to think about is eating. Or should you?

Nausea is individualistic—no single remedy is guaranteed to work for everyone, every time. But to judge how you're feeling and whether or not to try food, follow this simple advice.

If you're vomiting or feel like you're about to, don't eat or drink anything for a couple of hours, says Wanda Filer, M.D., a family physician in York, Pennsylvania. Your stomach is telling you that it needs some time to calm down.

When your stomach stops heaving, sip some flat soda, water, Gatorade-type fluid replacement, or chicken broth once or twice every five minutes. "But sip, don't gulp, so that the liquid has a chance to settle," says Dr. Filer.

Only when the nausea starts to level off or isn't that strong in the first place will eating help. Stick with small amounts of plain, low-fat foods like crackers, bananas, rice, applesauce, or dry toast.

If you're sick for more than three days or you frequently feel nauseated for no apparent reason, see a doctor. This is particularly true if you're also vomiting, experiencing abdominal pain, or losing weight unintentionally.

Drink Away Urinary Tract Infections

"Hydration is the best thing you can do for a UTI," says Kristene E. Whitmore, M.D., chief of urology at Graduate Hospital in Philadelphia.

"Drinking water is fashionable, it's good for you, and women whom I treat say that it's more effective than drug treatment."

Although a woman can have a UTI without knowing it, common signs and symptoms include pain and a burning sensation when urinating, urinating frequently, voiding just a few drops at a time, or passing blood in the urine.

Here's what you can do to relieve symptoms and prevent recurrences.

Fix yourself a baking soda cocktail. "At the first sign of symptoms, mix half a teaspoon of baking soda in an eight-ounce glass of water and drink it," says Dr. Whitmore. The baking soda raises the pH (acid/base balance) of irritating, acidic urine.

Get juiced. Drinking cranberry or blueberry juice cocktails can prevent bacteria from sticking to cells that line the urinary tract. Cranberry juice can act as an irritant in some women with urinary tract sensitivity, in which case Dr. Whitmore suggests diluting it.

Drink water on the hour. Drink one glass of water every hour for eight hours, enough so that your urine is clear. Drinking water helps dilute and flush out the bacteria that are trying to stick to the cells lining your urethra.

If you have more than two urinary tract infections (or what you think are urinary tract infections) in six months, or more than three episodes in a year, see a doctor, says Dr. Whitmore. And always consult a physician if you experience any of the following symptoms: blood in your urine, chills, nausea, vomiting, or lower-back pain.

part

8

Achieving
Optimum
Health:
A Man's
Guide

Making Sense of It All

It used to be that women took the lead in looking after their families' health—including the health of the men in their lives. Today, more guys are getting hip to good health. They're snuffing out their stogies, working off their spare tires, and reading up on everything from supplements to sexual potency.

Today, real men eat low-fat, high-fiber, for a whole host of reasons, as you'll read here: to prevent heart disease, obviously; for weight control, of course; and, yes, even to preserve their sexual health.

Who needs Viagra?!

New research reveals that for men, like women, there are many natural alternatives available to help us stay healthy and active into old age. Men over age 50, for example, will be relieved to hear that herbal treatments are showing promise as an alternative to surgery and potent prescription drugs for a common prostate problem called benign prostatic hyperplasia (BPH).

More food for thought: Read why the "love apple" may prevent prostate cancer and how one tablespoon of psyllium a day can counter the ill effects of a diet high in processed foods.

What's more, new gender-specific research (originally focused on women's health) is yielding life-saving recommendations for the gander as well as for the goose. Read why men need to take calcium requirements as seriously as women do. But beware of iron; while it might be just what the doctor ordered for her, extra iron can have serious (even life-threatening) consequences for him.

In what may be today's most important advice given to men, five renowned (male) physicians share their personal prescriptions for vitamin supplementation, stress management, heart health, alternative medicine, and sexual matters.

Finally, read how to "Beat Eight Sneaky Health Problems Guys Get" for tips on preventing common but unexpected health problems like gout, back pain, and inner-ear problems. Here are the best bets in natural healing for men and boys.

Positive Action Plans

Answers to Every Man's Questions about Supplements

For many of us, the premise is irresistible: Swallow this vitamin pill, it will make everything better. A day's worth of dietary shortcomings can vanish in a single gulp. One little capsule can shield us from ill health. Our energy will return; our hair will sprout; we'll be able to hypnotize women with our voices.

That's hard to swallow. If only it were that easy. Walk into a drugstore today, and you're faced with a mind-numbing array of choices: an alphabet soup of vitamins and a mother lode of minerals, available individually and in every possible combination. It's tempting to grab the closest bottle and head for the cashier.

But this is one decision that you don't want to make in the dark. Here's what some experts say about top-selling multivitamins.

Do I really need a multivitamin? Good question. While women of childbearing age have a host of jazzed-up nutrient needs, men generally don't. And men as a group risk fewer deficiencies than women do, simply because we eat more, according to Jeffrey Blumberg, Ph.D., professor of nutrition at Tufts University in Medford, Massachusetts. "If you're consuming 3,000 calories a day—even if you're eating pretty lousy—you'll still consume lots of vitamins and minerals," he says.

"Food is really where it's at, in terms of health protection," says Suzanne Hendrich, Ph.D., professor of food science and human nutrition at Iowa State University at Ames. "There's more to food than just vitamins and minerals, things like fiber and phytochemicals."

And the fact is, you may already be taking a multivitamin without knowing it. "If you're eating fortified cereal every morning, such as Total or Life, you don't need a supplement," says Paul Lachance, Ph.D., professor and chairman in the department of food science at Rutgers University in New Brunswick, New Jersey. In essence, experts say, Total is just a multivitamin in cereal form. Many energy bars also contain 100 percent of the RDA—the Recommended Dietary Allowance—for lots of vitamins and minerals.

That said, Dr. Hendrich concedes that a little insurance never hurt anybody. And even Dr. Blumberg admits that he pops a multivitamin/mineral supplement every day. The conclusion seems to be that a healthy diet is the most important part of your game plan; vitamins are your backups.

What should I look for? By definition, all nutrients are essential. But here are a handful that guys might be lacking in their diets, according to Dr. Blumberg: vitamins B_2, B_6, C, and E; folic acid; and the minerals selenium and chromium. Dr. Blumberg also suggests choosing a multi that gets at least some of its vitamin A as beta-carotene. "Beta-carotene is converted to vitamin A in the body, but it also has health benefits independent of vitamin A," he says. "Particularly in cancer prevention." Also, check for the following:

• *A reasonably short ingredients list.* "Things like PABA, inositol, bee pollen, and lecithin haven't been shown to be essential to human diets," says Marilyn Bush, C.N.S. (clinical nurse specialist), instructor of nutritional pharmacology at the University of Mississippi in Oxford. "Sometimes, ingredients are added simply to boost the price and make the product appear more complete."

• *Bushels of antioxidants.* "We're learning a lot about free radical formation and its relationship to heart disease and cancer," says Dr. Lachance. "So we're talking about the big killers, and many people are low on these antioxidants." Look for 250 milligrams of vitamin C, 200 milligrams of E, 3 milligrams or 5,000 international units (IU) of A as beta-carotene, and as much as 100 micrograms of selenium. If your multi has ballpark levels of these nutrients, you're covered.

• *No gimmicks.* For example, Dr. Blumberg says, there's no need for timed-release supplements. "Humans weren't designed to maintain a steady supply of vitamin C, or any other nutrient, throughout the day," he says. "There's no advantage in that."

• *An expiration date.* "They're still not universal," Dr. Blumberg says. "If one multi has an expiration date and one doesn't, which do you think I'd buy?"

Are name brands better than store brands? A bottle of Centrum multis goes for $6.54 for 60 tablets at a local drugstore, while the same quantity of a store brand costs three bucks. Is that extra three bucks worth it? Not necessarily. A generic brand that you trust is generally as good as the more expensive brand name. The reason is that a lot of the brand names and the store names are made by the same manufacturers. In any case, the Food and Drug Administration doesn't monitor multis with an iron grip, if you'll forgive the expression; it'll be a few years until standardized labels like those found on food products will be mandatory. And Dr. Blumberg says that soon, a nongovernment group called United States Pharmacopeia (USP) will put its seal of approval on multis that it deems acceptable. "But until that's universal and required, you can't know for sure that you're getting a quality product," he says. "The bottom line is, go with something you trust."

Are "natural" vitamins better somehow? Nah. In most cases, your body can't tell the difference between a vitamin or mineral that comes from food and one from a test tube. "Essentially, you get the same chemical structure," says Leon Ellenbogen, Ph.D., who works in nutritional sciences at Whitehall-Robins, maker of Centrum.

What's more, supplements labeled "natural" aren't necessarily safer, according to Dr. Hendrich. "Some of those 'natural' sources have higher levels of contaminants, such as lead, compared with the more carefully refined ingredients used in the manufacturing process," she says.

Do I need a "men's" multi? Most of the current crop of men's multis boast that they have no iron, so the real questions here is, "Should I avoid taking extra iron?" While some experts say that the RDA of 18 milligrams of supplemental iron is okay for men, most agree that that amount is overkill at best—and potentially dangerous at worst.

"Iron is a good example of why men shouldn't be taking women's supplements," says Dr. Lachance. "Men need to be careful with iron. If you're not anemic, you don't need it." He concedes that men who are strict vegetarians may need a bit of supplemental iron—but just a bit. "Eighteen milligrams is a lot of iron," he says. For men, Dr. Lachance recommends 10 milligrams daily as a maximum.

The bottom line is, look for a multi with 10 milligrams of iron. If you eat meat, forget it. You're getting plenty of iron.

Should I take "megadoses" of certain vitamins or minerals? No. Super-high levels of one nutrient may throw others out of balance, says Dr. Hendrich, and it's too easy to overdose with tablets of individual vitamins and minerals—which is why she recommends taking a multivitamin, rather than a shelf-full of single tablets. "Very large doses of iron, zinc, selenium, or manganese could carry some risks, from liver disease to neurological problems," she says. What's considered a "megadose"? For Dr. Hendrich, 10 times the DV for most vitamins is the absolute upper limit; for minerals, it's five times the DV. "In general, minerals have much greater toxic potential than vitamins," she explains. "But in any case, staying close to the DV is definitely a good idea."

Dr. Blumberg agrees that the vitamins aisle is no place to experiment. "It's important to note that five times the DV for vitamin E is safe. Yet take five times the DV for vitamin A, and you're risking toxicity." If you want to pop anything stronger than a balanced multivitamin/mineral supplement, consult your doctor first.

Beat Eight Sneaky Health Problems Guys Get

Weird things happen all the time. Tires blow out, lightning strikes, trains crash—and there's little we can do to prevent it. But we can help prevent some of the unexpected (and not-so-rare) health problems that strike many men. You already know about the importance of exercise, eating right, and getting regular checkups. But you might not know about these very simple steps that could save you a lot of pain—and maybe even save your life.

1. Walk to Borneo . . . or London. Airplane seats are starting to gain a nasty reputation for causing thromboses, or blood clots. It's no wonder: Sitting through *Mr. Holland's Opus* and a four-hour snooze will make blood pool in your legs. Blood that doesn't move can coagulate. Then, as you start walking again, clots can travel to the arteries that supply blood to your lungs.

"No one keeps statistics," says Stanley Mohler, M.D., director of aerospace medicine at Wright State University School of Medicine in Dayton, Ohio. "But clots probably occur at airports around the world every day." It happened to Dan Quayle in 1994, so it's not a Chicken Little worry. Take precautions: Drink a lot of nonalcoholic liquids. Dehydration caused by dry airplane air can cause blood platelets to clump. And of course, keep moving.

"Stroll around the cabin at least once, preferably twice, an hour," says Dr. Mohler. If you keep moving at about the same rate that you do at work, your capillaries should stay unplugged.

2. Take a tablespoon of psyllium every day. Eating powder made from psyllium plant seeds may sound a little strange, but it's one of the best ways to guard against diverticulitis. This painful condition occurs when weak spots in your intestinal lining bulge due to bowel pressure, like an inner tube ballooning through a hole in a tire. Particles collect in the pouches and cause infection. A recent study from the Hospital des Diaconesses in Paris found that diverticulitis is 10 times as common as it was a century ago. The main reason is that we're eating more processed foods.

Of course, adding more fiber to your diet is the answer. "The high-fiber diet of the South African Bantu allows them the lowest incidence of diverticulitis in the world," says Edward Goldberg, M.D., professor of gastroenterology at Lenox Hill Hospital in New York City. Great advice, but who eats their recommended 25 grams of fiber daily? Who even wants to think about it?

Psyllium is extremely high in fiber and is painless to eat. "A small daily serving can help prevent pouching of the intestinal lining," says Dr. Goldberg. So pick up some psyllium powder at any health food store and throw a tablespoon in your cereal or soup every day. It'll keep you in the clear.

3. Cut down your leg extensions. Major League catchers and middle-age men often have one thing in common: wrecked knees. Weak leg muscles and a shoddy foot-strike (from an orthopedic problem) can slowly pull the kneecap out of line. This causes the cartilage grinding that eventually leads to a painful condition called patellofemoral syndrome. "You'll probably feel it first as a sharp pain under your kneecap as you're climbing the stairs," says Allan Levy, M.D., team physician for the New York Giants.

If you've felt a twinge or two in your knees, the way to stave off further pain is to strengthen the muscles around your knee joint, says Dr. Levy. Do seated leg extensions, but only the top six to eight inches of the exercise. Simply mount a leg-extension machine, put the pin on a light weight, and straighten your legs. Bend your knees slightly, and then press the pad back to the top. Ten repetitions three times a week should do it. "If you go through the bottom part of the exercise, you'll grind your kneecap more," warns Dr. Levy. Drugstore orthotic inserts may also help correct the way your foot lands, but talk to your doctor. Knee grinding also can speed up osteoarthritis.

4. Keep your neck straight. If you picked up a nasty neck crick after a day in the gym, it probably wasn't from that 180-pound shoulder press that you foolishly attempted. It was most likely a sloppy set of crunches, says Stephen Hochschuler, M.D., chairman of the Texas Back Institute in Plano. Pulling your head can stress the neck joints, which makes supporting your 12-pound brain box painful. Keep your hands on your chest and don't tuck your chin during situps, warns Dr. Hochschuler. "Imagine that you're holding a softball between your chin and chest," he advises.

Neck pain can be caused by bicycling, as well. The problem can be a low seat or low handlebars, either of which can force you to arch your neck. Head to a local bike shop for proper adjustments.

5. Skip high-protein diets. Bodybuilders, dinosaurs, and other clumsy carnivores who eat too much protein can end up walking funny. It's not from going barefoot, it's from gout. Gout is a common male disorder that causes pain in the knuckle of your big toe and other joints. Though it's hereditary, it can be spurred by high blood pressure and diabetes. It was called the rich-man's disease because it often results from a diet of red meat, fish, pâté, and alcohol. These high-protein foods create uric acid crystals, which become wedged in your lowest joints—typically, your wrists, knees, and toes. After a while, the gritty crystals cause painful inflammation. "The pain is so great that some people can't stand to have bedsheets resting on their toes," says David Goldfarb, M.D., co-director of the kidney stone prevention and treatment program at New York University Medical Center in New York City.

Gout usually hits men older than age 60, but you can nip it now. Keep your protein intake less than 20 percent of your diet and take a blood test for uric acid during your next physical. High levels don't necessarily guarantee that you'll develop gout, but it's fair warning to change your diet. If joint pain has already struck, ask your doctor about anti-arthritic drugs.

6. Pop an antihistamine. We've all felt pressure in our ears while flying or scuba diving. Few of us, however, know that it can damage our hearing. Hold your nose, close your mouth, and gently blow. If your ears don't "pop" within a few seconds, you may have eustachian tube dysfunction, according to Christopher Linstrom, M.D., chief of otology at the

New York Eye and Ear Infirmary in New York City. That means the valves that clear ear pressure are blocked, and sudden changes in pressure could actually injure your delicate inner ear.

According to researchers at the Gentofte University Hospital in Denmark, an estimated 5 percent of adult flyers (and 25 percent of children) suffer from such ear problems. Luckily, they're preventable.

"Tube dysfunction is often associated with allergies," says Dr. Linstrom. "Antihistamines that bring down sinus swelling usually open the tubes." Taking an antihistamine (choose one that won't cause drowsiness) prior to flying or diving may allow you to equalize faster. If the problem is chronic, an otologist can insert a tube in your ear that will relieve the pressure.

7. Nip colon cancer in the bud. If you're older than 40, ask your doctor to test for hidden blood in your stool during your exam. This simple screening test can decrease your risk of colon cancer, says Cary Schneebaum, M.D., a gastroenterologist at Beth Israel Hospital in New York City.

Blood in the bowels usually means one of two things: hemorrhoids or polyps, growths on the wall of the colon that may become cancerous. A study at Oregon Health Sciences University in Portland, of 297 patients with rectal bleeding, 26 had polyps and 13 had colon cancer. Colon cancer almost always starts as polyps, so removing them early can prevent it. Case closed.

Heed the other warnings between exams, says Dr. Schneebaum. Head to your doctor if you have persistent abdominal cramps, constant diarrhea or constipation, or—of course—if you see red in your stool.

8. Stretch before you swing. Elton Strauss, M.D., chief of orthopaedic trauma at Mount Sinai Medical Center in New York City, sees many weekend golfers who have agonizing lower-back pain because they didn't follow a very simple warm-up plan before teeing off. The twisting motion of a golf swing can strain the muscles that attach the pelvis to the thigh, says Dr. Strauss. "You'll know when you've done it," he says. "The pain centers right under the belt line over the gluteal region." That is, a pain in the butt.

A little stretching can save you months of discomfort, says Dr. Strauss. Walk at a fast clip to warm up, then touch your toes with your knees bent to flex your spine. Finish by gently twisting your body with your hands on your hips. In five minutes, you're ready to drive.

Advice That (Male) Doctors Live By

The world is full of impostors, people who say one thing and do another. Is there anybody out there who talks the talk and walks the walk?

There's definitely something to learn from legitimate authorities who not only know what they're talking about but also practice what they preach. Here's advice from some of them, including a 65-year-old heart doctor who has beaten a family history of cardiovascular disease, and an energetic urologist who is more satisfied with his sexual performance at age 46 than he was at 26. These men have been so impressed with what they've learned that they're living the lessons. If the ultimate endorsement of something is to make it your own, then their tips constitute the perfect prescription. Here's how some of America's top docs stay healthy. Any of their strategies can work for you.

On Vitamin Supplements

Mark Levine, M.D., chief of the molecular and clinical nutrition center at the National Institutes of Health, is an expert on vitamins and minerals and their impact on health, yet you won't find a bottle of Centrum or One-a-Day in his medicine cabinet. Instead, he prefers to swallow his essential nutrients by eating five or more servings of fruits and vegetables daily.

"For people who can't or won't do that, then a multivitamin supplement is okay," he explains. "But I find it easiest to eat fruits and vegetables. The best data say that fruits and vegetables are protective against disease. But what is it exactly that's protective? Is it vitamin C? Is it one of the B vitamins? Is it folate? Is it lycopene, carotenoid, or something totally unknown? Or is it a combination of everything? No one knows. The bottom line is, the data say that the benefits come from fruits and vegetables, so they're what I eat."

Dr. Levine manages this by keeping bananas, grapes, oranges, and different kinds of seasonal produce handy. There might be a bunch of bananas on his desk, some grapes in a drawer, or an orange in the office refrigerator. When he's hungry, they're within easy, effortless reach. "There are so many choices," he adds. "All you have to do is think about it a bit and plan."

The 45-year-old Dr. Levine does supplement his diet by drinking two glasses of skim milk daily for the calcium ("Men forget that they need it as much as women do") and by taking 200 international units (IU) of vitamin E to reduce his risk of heart attack. (Vitamin E is a powerful antioxidant naturally present in fatty nuts and oils.)

"I don't have enough vitamin E in my diet," he explains, "so I take it as a supplement to minimize my risk of cardiovascular disease. There's no definitive evidence that it does this, but the potential benefit is there, and I don't see any harm in that dosage."

Dr. Levine emphasizes, however, that it takes more than these magical ingredients to stay healthy and live long. It takes a combination of low-fat eating, prudent living, exercising, and controlling weight. (He can still fit in his high school suit.) Although most Americans would like to believe otherwise, he says that there's no miracle supplement that can make up for deficiencies in these areas.

On Sexual Potency

At 46, an age when many men are already troubled by flagging sex drives or occasional impotence, Irwin Goldstein, M.D., urologist at Boston University Medical Center, says that he has never encountered any significant problems and is, in fact, enjoying sex more now than he did in his twenties.

"The few bouts of impotence that I have experienced have been related to alcohol use," he says. "It's a really bad drug to have on board. If I go to a party and see some guys loading down the drinks, I know that their evening afterward will be very predictable."

Dr. Goldstein attributes his sexual health to the following five pillars of potency, tenets that he preaches in his lectures and practices in his private life.

I keep my endothelial cells healthy. These cells form the internal lining of all the blood vessels in your body. It's believed that any injury to them can lead to plaque deposits that cause the narrowing of arteries and heart disease. Unrestricted blood flow is vital not only to cardiovascular health but also to sexual health. Blood makes your penis firm and delivers a fresh supply of nourishing oxygen. Without it, you'd resemble an overripe grape withering on the vine.

Dr. Goldstein scrubs his endothelials by eating a low-fat, high-fiber diet and exercising regularly (situps, stairclimbing, walking). "It's all pretty straightforward stuff that most physicians will tell you about living your life," he says. "But a unique way to look at it is that you're only as healthy as these endothelial cells, and you'll age only as quickly as they do."

I never ride a bicycle. Dr. Goldstein doesn't trust bikes, because their seats force you to support much of your weight on the soft tissue between your pelvic bones. Since this nether region contains nerves and arteries that feed the penis, any pressure that's exerted for long periods can have serious consequences. One of Dr. Goldstein's patients, for example, became impotent from regularly riding a stationary bike. Horseback riding or straddling any narrow seat can do similar damage. "I never sit on anything where my legs are spread and my body weight is on my crotch," he states.

I'm careful during coitus. "During sexual intercourse, I'm very careful not to bend, twist, spindle, or mutilate," says Dr. Goldstein. "Penises in the erect state are very vulnerable to injury. They're not designed to bear the weight of a full-grown female on top of you."

I have erections often. "In the flaccid state, the penis receives less than 0.1 percent of the blood circulating through the body," says Dr. Goldstein. "That's lower than virtually every other organ. Its oxygen level is also very low, 35 millimeters of mercury compared with 55 to 60 in most organs. The only time when the penis gets a lot of blood and oxygen is during erections. Hence the saying, 'Use it or lose it.' Erections recharge your batteries."

You can accomplish this with frequent sex and masturbation or, if you're not as blessed or don't want to regress, a simple good night's sleep. "You typically have 1½ to 3 hours of penile erection during a normal, healthy night's sleep," he explains. He warns, however, that some antidepressants and certain sleeping pills can diminish the deep phases of sleep, when this natural rejuvenation occurs.

I know to treat any erection problem quickly. Don't handle erectile dysfunction as you would a head cold, waiting patiently for it to clear. "It's far smarter to get treatment earlier rather than later," says Dr. Goldstein. "If your penis isn't getting the oxygen that it needs, mild impotence can easily become serious impotence, and then many of the newer, noninvasive therapies won't be useful."

On Heart Health

The Framingham Heart Study is the longest continuous investigation of heart disease ever conducted. Begun in 1948, it has provided new insight into the workings of the most mysterious muscle in our bodies and has contributed to the declining incidence of heart disease in America. *Prevention* heart disease advisor William Castelli, M.D., medical director of the Framingham, Massachusetts, Cardiovascular Institute, former director of the Framingham Heart Study, and a cardiologist and epidemiologist who has been involved with the project since the mid-1960s, has learned its lessons and taken them to heart.

"One day, years ago, when we were going over the reports, I noticed that the average cholesterol count of the men in the study who had suffered heart attacks was around 240 (mg/dl, or milligrams per deciliter)," he recalls. "My cholesterol at the time was about 270. (In those days, 300+ was considered the danger zone. So I suddenly said to myself, if these guys are dropping dead and they all had cholesterol lower than mine, then what makes me think my cholesterol count is so good?"

Compounding this fear was Dr. Castelli's family history. Then in his mid-thirties, he knew that his family had a "terrible history of heart disease," plus he was already wearing a spare tire around his middle. So he decided to make an experiment of himself, and has continued, with the following plan.

I eat more fiber. "I start every day with a big bowl of rolled oats," he explains, "to which I add an equal amount of applesauce or nonfat yogurt. It gives me a great dose of soluble fiber, which has been shown in about 37 studies to lower cholesterol and heart attack rates."

I reduce saturated-fat intake to less than 10 grams per day. "I cut out butter, fatty beef, hot dogs, and high saturated fat cheeses," he says. But he didn't totally eliminate the foods that he loves. Rather, he searched for more healthful alternatives. For example, he found a Vermont Cheddar that has 75 percent less saturated fat, 98 percent fat-free filet mignons from a ranch in South Dakota and, of late, low-fat hot dogs.

I eat fish often. "I eat grilled fish about five times a week," says Dr. Castelli. The omega-3 fatty acids that it contains have been shown to prevent arteriosclerosis. "We give fish oil to all our patients who have extremely high triglycerides."

I eat lots of fruits and vegetables. "I eat at least five servings a day," he says. "Most of these come at lunch when I eat an extremely large salad. Two vegetables and a smaller salad with dinner round out the day. I snack on fruit."

I drink alcohol moderately. Whether it's wine, beer, or whiskey, Dr.

Castelli points out, having one alcoholic drink per day (no more) lowers heart disease risk and even the threat of death from cancer. If you can't tolerate alcohol, however, don't start drinking, he advises. You don't want to replace one risk with another. "I love red wine," he adds. "I generally buy a nice bottle and make it last one week."

I take supplements. "I take 400 IU of vitamin E, 200 micrograms of selenium, and 200 micrograms of chromium every day because there are good clinical trials showing their effectiveness in fighting heart disease," he says. "I also take folic acid and 81 milligrams of enteric-coated aspirin daily."

I exercise to raise "good" cholesterol. "I jog about 15 miles a week, usually three five-mile runs," explains Dr. Castelli. "Each one of the runs usually takes about an hour. I've been doing this since the late 1970s, and my ratio of total cholesterol to HDL (high-density lipoprotein, the good kind) has improved dramatically."

I control stress. "The best ways that I've found are to pray, and to never ask yourself how you're doing. You'll never be young, pretty, handsome, popular, or rich enough, so don't try."

So what has been the result of all these changes? "Now, my cholesterol is under 200," he boasts, "and at age 65, I've outdistanced both my brother and my father—by more than 25 years—in staying free of cardiovascular disease. I'm convinced that it's because I've led a prudent lifestyle."

On Stress Management

Paul J. Rosch, M.D., clinical professor of medicine and psychiatry at New York Medical College in Valhalla, is in his early seventies. When he goes to conferences and leaves his office for a week, the paperwork piles up—as it does for most executives. But instead of exhibiting high-stress symptoms, Dr. Rosch has found ways to avoid getting overworked.

"There's only a certain amount that I can do," says Dr. Rosch, "so I prioritize." When he returns from a conference, he separates the paperwork into three piles—work that must be done immediately, work that's important but can wait, and a third pile composed of work that isn't as important and can wait longer. "I try to take control of the situation and, if necessary, be willing to say no."

The main technique that Dr. Rosch, a stress researcher for more than 40 years, uses to minimize stress in his life is to work at a job that he loves. Typically, job stress stems from laboring at an occupation where you have little influence over or pride in the final product. Unlike our ancestors who worked farms or ran taverns, modern-day laborers are used to an assembly-line process. Dr. Rosch, though, has been able to retain a bit of that bygone expertise and single-handed craftsmanship in his position as president of the American Institute of Stress in Yonkers, New York.

"You often see this with symphony conductors or entertainers who would appear to be under lots of stress by having to cope with arduous travel schedules and prima donnas," he explains. "Yet they live long, healthy lives. People like George Burns or Bob Hope, for example. The reason is because they're involved in altruistic egotism—doing something that they enjoy and that benefits others. It's a powerful stress buster, as is having a strong social support system with lots of friends. I've been fortunate in this regard."

Dr. Rosch is adamant, however, that stress is a highly individualized thing. What he finds pleasurable, others might find distressing. And everyone needs some degree of stress in his life to be healthy and productive. "It's very much like the tension on a violin string," he explains. "If you don't have enough tension, the violin will play a dull, raspy note. If you have too much, there will be a shrill, shrieking sound or the string will snap. But just the right amount creates a beautiful tone. We all have to find the right amount of stress in our lives that allows us to make beautiful music."

On Alternative Medicines

Seventy-year-old herb expert and *Prevention* advisor Varro E. Tyler, Ph.D., Sc.D., describes himself as an "old-time pharmacist," who is naturally skeptical of many overhyped New Age cures. At the same time, he realizes the simple wisdom of certain natural treatments as a first line of defense.

When he feels a cold or flu building, for example, the first thing he does is swallow an echinacea capsule. He then continues taking this herb until the symptoms fade. "It won't kill the virus or the bacteria," he explains, "but it will stimulate the immune system," which often shortens the duration of the illness and minimizes symptoms.

When Dr. Tyler suffers indigestion or gas, he brews some chamomile tea. "It has both an anti-inflammatory and an antispasmodic effect, so it relaxes the stomach muscles and helps me feel better." Although he buys his chamomile in an herb market to ensure potency, he says that commercial tea is fine if steeped for 15 minutes in a covered pot. "The oil in chamomile isn't very water soluble," he explains, "so you have to make sure that it dissolves as much as possible."

Surprisingly, these are the only two herbal remedies that Dr. Tyler uses regularly. If he had high cholesterol, he says, he'd take garlic tablets. "The beneficial, cholesterol-fighting compound in garlic is called allicin, but cooking destroys much of it," he explains, "so it's better either to eat raw garlic, and risk losing some friends, or to take it in an odorless capsule form." Make sure that the label of the brand you're buying lists allicin either as an ingredient or as a by-product ("allicin yield"). "The best-selling garlic preparation in the United States doesn't contain any allicin," he notes.

If Dr. Tyler was bothered by migraine headaches, he says, he'd reach for an herbal product called feverfew and take 125 milligrams every day. If he suffered from insomnia, at bedtime he'd take a capsule of valerian, a plant root that has been used as a sleeping aid for 2,000 years and "is much more proven in terms of safety than melatonin, which has been on the market only a short time."

Finally, if Dr. Tyler hadn't had his prostate removed five years ago because of a malignancy, he'd probably be taking saw palmetto to reduce inflammation of the gland and minimize nocturnal bathroom visits. "I think it's as effective as any prescription drug currently on the market in this country," he adds.

And what does Dr. Tyler say to skeptics who argue that the effectiveness of these remedies is all in the minds of the users? "Certainly, the placebo effect is well-documented," he explains. "But it works only about a third of the time, so people need to face reality. In the herbal field, this is hard to do because there's so much hyperbole and unproven information. But there is a sound nucleus of research for a couple dozen remedies that shows them to be truly useful and relatively free of side effects. In many cases, they should be tried before more potent medicines. Take them only when you have to, though. That's been my philosophy throughout my life."

How to Find an Alternative Therapist

More and more Americans are seeking information on all kinds of alternative therapies, from acupuncture and homeopathy to biofeedback and massage. But identifying the therapies that offer the most hope for your problems is just the beginning. If you want to pursue alternative health care, you'll need to find a qualified practitioner.

But how?

"I'll tell you how I used to find them," offers James Gordon, M.D., professor of psychiatry and family medicine at Georgetown University in Washington, D.C. These days, the good doctor needs no such help: Chairman of the first advisory board of the National Institutes of Health's Office of Alternative Medicine, Dr. Gordon is currently director of the Center for Mind/Body Medicine in Washington, D.C., where both he and his patients have no problem obtaining referrals to the area's top alternative practitioners. But it was not always like this. Years ago, Dr. Gordon traveled around the country a lot. Troubled by a bad back, he would often find himself in terrible pain in a strange city where he knew no one. What did he do?

"I'd find out where the best local health food store was, go there, and ask the staff, 'Who's the best person in the area who does manipulation for back pain?' I always found someone good—a chiropractor, an osteopath trained in manipulation, sometimes a massage therapist."

In some cases, the best sources are professional organizations that represent each therapy's practitioners. Sometimes, the information is available with a single phone call, though some organizations require a small check before they'll send out listings. Often, the best, most complete information is available on the World Wide Web—free.

Also, the Office of Alternative Medicine (OAM) at the National Institutes of Health, although they don't make actual referrals, can send you information. Write and request their "General Information Package." It includes good advice on locating and selecting an alternative care practitioner. Contact the OAM Clearinghouse, P.O. Box 8218, Silver Spring, MD 20907.

Here's a sampling of all the resources available to help you locate the right alternative health care practitioner for you.

Your Family Doctor

You may think of your family physician as only a source of Western medicine. But the truth, says Dr. Gordon, is that "he is probably more open to alternative therapies than you would expect."

Medical studies back this view. For instance, a University of Maryland at Baltimore survey of 180 family physicians found that 54 percent had used biofeedback in their practices, 35 percent had used massage therapy, more than 56 percent had referred their patients to a chiropractor, and more than 27 percent referred patients to an acupuncturist or a hypnotist. "It becomes clear," the researchers note, "that some therapies previously considered alternative are now viewed as part of mainstream medicine."

These open-minded family doctors are probably the most underutilized resource to alternative medicine. *The New England Journal of Medicine* reported that the vast majority—72 percent—of people who used "unconventional medical therapies" did not even tell their doctors about it, much less ask for referrals. This, despite the fact that almost everyone who saw an alternative care practitioner for a serious medical condition was also being treated by a "regular" doctor. So ask your family doc first.

Other Connections

But what if your doctor doesn't know whom to send you to?

"Friends are the best place to start," says Dr. Gordon, "because they want to help you—and they know you, so they should have a good sense of who would work well with you. Ask family members, or ask at the health food store, like I did," says Dr. Gordon. "The people who work there are often very connected to the area's best practitioners."

And don't limit yourself to your area. "Call everyone until you find someone who knows a practitioner they think is great," suggests Adriane Fugh-Berman, M.D., chairwoman of the National Women's Health Network, an independent consumer advocacy organization in Washington, D.C.; nationally recognized authority on alternative medicine; and author of the book *Alternative Medicine: What Works.* "Have them ask that person if there's anyone in your area whom they'd recommend. A lot of practitioners know their peers in other areas of the country," she explains.

Support groups can be another great source of practitioner referrals, notes Dr. Gordon, especially when you're seeking help for a specific condition. But such groups are just like doctors, he warns; there are good and bad, so be selective. "Stay away from groups that wallow in self-pity and depression," he advises, "and be cautious if they seem to advocate only one type of therapy—conventional or alternative."

Ask your doctor or local hospital for the names of support groups in your area or look for them on the World Wide Web. Then make some phone calls and, if possible, attend one of their local meetings. "Ask group members about practitioners they've had experience with," he suggests.

Referral Resource

For any given alternative—or conventional—medical discipline, there's at least one organization that you can contact for information. Many are well-equipped to refer you to practitioners in your area—particularly if you have access to online information and you can access World Wide Web home pages maintained by those organizations.

Accessible and easy to use, the Web sites provide lots of great information about licensing, certification, and the therapy itself. Most of the sites have a list of practitioners that you can access via a variety of categories, such as city (best if you live in or near a major one), Zip code (identifies practitioners that share your first three digits—great for well-populated areas that aren't necessarily big cities), and state (for folks in those small ones, where the names on the maps have to float out in the ocean).

If you're not "wired" and none of your friends are online, your local library may have Internet access.

How to Choose

Although the lists provided by some organizations are just names and addresses, others offer additional information. The list of homeopathic practitioners, for instance, includes each member's abbreviated medical profession designation (M.D., D.O., N.D., PA-C) and a two-page explanation of what all those initials mean (so you'll know, for instance, that a PA-C is a physician's assistant who's certified in that field).

Many of the lists also indicate when someone works out of a clinic or group practice, where you would likely have a choice of practitioners—and maybe even a choice of alternative therapies—at a single location.

Here are a few other tips for choosing the right individual.

Define your needs. "Are you just trying to take better care of yourself, or do you need help for a specific condition?" asks Dr. Gordon. "If it's the former, you'll want someone who can function as your primary care provider—maybe a naturopath or osteopath. If it's the latter, do some reading to learn which of the various therapies are thought to work best for certain conditions—like chiropractic or manipulative osteopathy for back pain, or acupuncture or massage for muscle pain."

But if you don't have any kind of primary care health professional, Dr. Gordon says, find that person first. "He can be an M.D., a naturopath, whatever—the important thing is that you have someone who will evaluate you and then monitor the care you get from others," he says.

Make a phone call. "A lot of publications suggest that you 'interview' a prospective health care provider before making a first appointment. A lot of professionals honestly don't have the time," notes Dr. Fugh-Berman. But, she suggests, you can always call the office staff with specific questions about the practice: How long is a typical first visit and how much does it cost? Is there a sliding fee scale for people with limited income? Will health insurance cover any portion of this care? What are the practitioner's credentials—is he state licensed or certified by a professional organization? Does he carry malpractice insurance?

"Organize your questions in advance," says Dr. Fugh-Berman, "and then see how you feel about the responses. Just be aware that you'll never be able to do enough advance work to be sure that a practitioner is perfect for you; eventually, you simply have to pick someone and go see him. And if you're still not happy after your visit, see someone else."

Know what you want. Think about the kind of care that you need and the type of people you work best with before that first visit, suggests Dr. Fugh-Berman. "Specifically, do you want someone who will be your health care partner, or do you prefer a health care professional who just tells you what to do? Not everyone who seeks out alternative care wants to make choices on his own or even be a part of the process—some people feel that being offered choices means that the practitioner doesn't know what to do." There's no right or wrong way—do what works for you.

Perhaps most important, trust your own judgment and instincts. "Just as you are often the best judge of what's wrong with your body," says Dr. Gordon, "you're usually the best judge of whether a practitioner is right for you."

Sage Advice

Heart of a Mad Man

He says he never loses his temper. She points out that he breaks a club across his knee every time he misses the rotating clown at Big Ed's Mini Golf. What's happening here isn't just a difference of opinion—it could be a tip-off that he's at risk for heart disease.

Most people probably know that mad is bad, heart-wise. But denying anger may be worse. Mark Ketterer, Ph.D., clinical psychologist at Henry Ford Hospital in Detroit, studied 144 men being treated for heart disease. He also polled each man's wife or significant other. Denial of anger—claiming to be a lamb when your partner pegs you as an irritable lion—was a stronger predictor of death or future heart problems than was any other risk factor, including hypertension (high blood pressure), diabetes, smoking, and anger itself.

"People who fail to acknowledge their distress may have difficulty returning to normal after they're angered," Dr. Ketterer explains, "without solving whatever problem is punching their buttons." So a short-term problem becomes chronic. Future research should clarify the impact of anger denial on people who don't already have heart disease, and on women. In the meantime, he suggests that spouses clue doctors in on their partners' moods. "If it were up to me, getting a report from the patient's significant other would be routine," Ketterer says.

Back Off, Jack: Dominance May Do You In

Constantly interrupting people may be considered rude and annoying, but hardly life-threatening. Yet a study of more than 700 men found that those who tended to interrupt, finish others' sentences, and try to take control of the conversation during an interview were 60 percent more likely to die during the next 22 years than were their non-domineering peers. "That's a considerable risk—about the same as someone who smokes half a pack of cigarettes a day," says study author Michael Babyak, Ph.D., of Duke University Medical Center in Durham, North Carolina.

What makes this behavior, which psychologists call social dominance, deadly is that it springs from super-competitiveness. "These are guys who always need to have it their way. That's a difficult thing to achieve, and it takes a constant flow of stress hormones for them to constantly assert themselves," Dr. Babyak explains. "For men, this chronic stress is hard on the body, particularly the heart and the arteries." (Women's health doesn't seem to be affected by social dominance, perhaps because of hormonal differences or differences in how women express dominance.)

Luckily, most men can learn to put less bite in their barks. If you treat conversation like combat, Dr. Babyak suggests taking a deep breath, counting to 10, or doing whatever is necessary to pause and ask yourself, "Do I really need to dominate here?" Some might benefit from relaxation techniques, but awareness is most of the battle.

Not that you have to turn from Superman into Clark Kent permanently. "In some cases, like in work situations or sports, competition is necessary or fun," says Dr. Babyak. The key is to remember that there's no Super Bowl for conversation.

Salsa Can Get to a Guy

You've heard that American men who eat more tomatoes and tomato products like salsa also get less prostate cancer. The reasons why aren't known yet. But scientists suspect a natural tomato compound called lycopene (tomatoes have lots; most foods don't). For the first time, an ultra-high analysis at Dana-Farber Cancer Institute in Boston has identified lycopene in samples of prostate tissue from 25 men. Not proof, yet, that lycopene protects the prostate. But proof that at least it gets there. Makes tomatoes (and salsa) look smarter than ever, guys.

Men and Their Bones: Some Hard Facts

Many men believe that osteoporosis—weakening of the skeleton due to bone loss—is exclusively the province of women. Not so, say experts. Men are at risk, too, and need to take action to keep their bones strong. Here are the facts.

- American men over age 50 have a greater chance of breaking a bone due to osteoporosis than they have of developing prostate cancer.
- Only about 1 out of 10 American men knows how much calcium is recommended to help keep bones strong (up to age 64, you need 1,000 milligrams a day; at age 65 and above, you need 1,500 milligrams a day).
- Only 4 out of 10 men actually get that much calcium in an average day.

Herbal Elixirs

Promising Herbs for Prostate Problems

Many men past age 50 suffer from benign prostatic hyperplasia. Here, herb expert and Prevention *advisor Varro E. Tyler, Ph.D., Sc.D., describes the herbs that may prove to be reasonable alternatives to surgery and drugs.*

The lovely nights of undisturbed sleep that you had looked forward to when the last of the kids packed up for college have not materialized. Instead, you find yourself logging half a dozen trips to the bathroom before dawn.

Chances are, you have a condition common in older men, called benign prostatic hyperplasia (BPH). That's when the prostate gland enlarges and partially obstructs the urethra, the tube that carries urine from the bladder. This results in an increased frequency of urination, accompanied by a frustrating inability to empty the bladder completely as well as problems with starting and stopping. A weaker urine stream may also be noticed.

Benign prostatic hyperplasia is very common in men over age 50. But before beginning any form of treatment, see your family doctor or a urologist for a professional diagnosis to rule out other more serious, but less common, conditions, such as cancer, that can cause similar complaints.

Once your doctor determines that BPH is the culprit, you'll discuss treatment options, including surgery and various types of prescription drugs. While all of these are more or less effective, they can also present undesirable side effects—most notably, impotence.

But before you resign yourself to frequent nighttime trips to the bathroom, or a diminished sex life, talk to your doctor about the many herbal products now being used for BPH. Here's a list of the most popular, including their track records.

Saw palmetto (*Serenoa repens*): most helpful

Of all the herbal treatments for BPH, the most promising, and certainly the most popular in the United States, is saw palmetto. Its effectiveness is supported by clinical studies from Europe, it is relatively free of side effects, and it's inexpensive.

The therapy involves the use of a fatty extract prepared from the ripe fruits of a native Florida palm tree known as saw palmetto, or sabal. Nearly all of the studies conducted in the past two decades, including one three-year trial, found statistically significant improvements in typical BPH symptoms. More than half of these studies were of the highest research standards. The results seen with saw palmetto were comparable to those achieved with the more commonly prescribed synthetic drugs. Side effects were limited primarily to stomach upsets.

How much to take? The recommended dose is 1 to 2 grams of the crude drug or 320 milligrams of an extract daily for the treatment of early stages of BPH, according to the German Commission E, the world's leading authority on herbal medicine. There are no known contraindications.

Pygeum (*Pygeums africanum*): most helpful

Second to saw palmetto is the powdered bark of pygeum, an evergreen tree native to southern and central Africa, which has long been used

Can Cranberry Concentrate Shrink an Enlarged Prostate?

Despite some claims to the contrary, cranberry juice or concentrate has no direct effect on the size of the prostate, nor does it have an anti-inflammatory effect on the tissue of that gland.

However, cranberry juice may help relieve urinary tract infections associated with benign prostatic hyperplasia (BPH). By preventing complete emptying of the bladder, BPH contributes to urinary retention and an increased risk of infection.

Compounds in cranberries called anti-adhesins help prevent infectious bacteria from sticking to the cells that line the urinary tract. As little as three ounces a day of cranberry juice cocktail—or an equivalent quantity of cranberry concentrate in capsules—is considered effective in preventing recurring infections. Unfortunately, cranberry is not particularly useful in treating full-blown infections. Prescription drugs are better for that.

there for urinary problems. European studies have established the effectiveness of the herb in treating BPH. During the past 20 years, 26 clinical trials—nearly half of them meeting rigorous scientific standards—were conducted with pygeum extract in about 600 patients. The results showed significant improvement in symptoms of BPH.

How much to take? The studies used a lipid extract of the bark in doses of 100 to 200 milligrams per day. But because Commission E has not examined pygeum, they have issued no judgment regarding its safety or efficacy. Toxicity tests in small animals in Europe turned up no serious side effects. The extract has been found to be well-tolerated throughout long-term administration.

Stinging nettle (*Urtica dioica*): might help

Another popular BPH treatment involves an extract prepared from the root of the common stinging nettle. Although 10 studies have been done on its effect on BPH, only 2 of those trials met the most exacting scientific standards. Both of those showed significant increases in urinary output, but urine flow remained unchanged, and the men were still unable to empty their bladders completely. Side effects included mild gastrointestinal complaints.

How much to take? Commission E has approved nettle root for the treatment of early stages of BPH at a daily dose equivalent to four to six grams of crude drug. In my opinion, the effectiveness of nettle root is by no means as well-proven as that of saw palmetto or pygeum.

Pumpkin seeds (*Cucurbita pepo*): questionable

Pumpkin seeds have long been used in folk medicine for the treatment of BPH. Presumably, the fatty oil and various other components have some beneficial effect on the condition, but studies to support this claim are almost entirely lacking. Nevertheless, a 1985 report with recommendations from Commission E authorized the administration of 10 grams of the seeds daily for early stages of BPH. Based on the lack of evidence, I question its effectiveness.

Beware the Love Potion

Yohimbe, from the dried bark of the African tree *Pausinystalia yohimbe*, has an ancient reputation as an aphrodisiac. Whatever effect the herb has is due to a mixture of alkaloids, of which the compound yohimbine is considered the most active.

Several clinical studies have suggested that yohimbine may be useful in treating erectile difficulties in males, especially those that are not related to physical factors such as nerve damage or surgery. Despite this, use of the herb, which is widely available in health food stores, cannot be recommended because of potential adverse side effects, such as agitation, tremors, anxiety, high blood pressure, rapid heartbeat, nausea, and vomiting. For this reason (and because of the fact that yohimbe's efficacy remains debatable) the herb has not been approved for use by the German Commission E, the world's leading authority on herbal medicine.

One more downside is that there's a 50-50 chance that the yohimbe product that you purchase will be worthless. In 1995, scientists analyzed 26 commercial yohimbe preparations. Nine of them didn't contain any yohimbine, and eight contained only trace amounts—not even close to the doses that may prove effective.

If you're experiencing impotence, see your physician. There is a prescription version of yohimbine that may help, and your doctor can monitor any side effects.

Home Remedies

Feed Your Sexual Appetite

With all the hype over Viagra, many men have been wondering whether there's a natural alternative—some kind of home remedy—that would help out older men. While there's no magic bullet, some natural aphrodisiacs have been used for many years.

Oysters have long boasted a kind of sex appeal, and for good reason. They're loaded with zinc, which is linked to fertility, potency, sex drive, and long-term sexual health. The mineral is critical to sperm production, and low zinc stores have been blamed for decreases in semen volume and testosterone levels, explains Sara Brewer, M.D., author of *Better Sex*. "Each ejaculation can expend up to five milligrams of zinc, or one-third of your daily allowance," Dr. Brewer says. Luckily, zinc is easy to come by. Four ounces of lean beef provides half the daily requirement, and a single oyster gives you the whole shebang. Turkey, cereal, and beans are other good sources.

But perhaps the biggest boost to sexual health is cholesterol-lowering foods, such as oatmeal, oat bran, dried beans, and any fruit with a peel. Cholesterol can clog your arteries, after all, including the ones that allow your penis to stand tall. For that reason, it's also a good idea to avoid cholesterol raisers like fried foods, butter, and red meat.

Help for a Hangover

While folk remedies for hangovers are more common than empty beer cans at a fraternity party, they're just about as useful, too, say experts.

So what should you do if you want to trump a hangover? The best you can do, experts say, is drink plenty of water (since alcohol tends to dehydrate you) and weather the storm.

If you want to try something else, though, try a drink such as spicy V-8 vegetable juice or even a virgin Bloody Mary, says Paul Lachance, Ph.D., professor and chairman in the department of food science at Rutgers University in New Brunswick, New Jersey. "Too much alcohol can create free radicals," he says, "and tomato juice and vegetable juice are good sources of antioxidants." Also, says Dr. Lachance, spices can help dilate blood vessels, which could speed recovery by improving blood circulation to your throbbing head.

One final note: Stay away from acetaminophen (the painkiller found in Tylenol) before, during, or after a night of drinking. Acetaminophen with alcohol makes a dangerous combination that can lead to liver damage, says David Whitcomb, M.D., Ph.D., of the University of Pittsburgh Medical Center. "Doses up to two grams—about four Extra-Strength Tylenol—are probably okay," he says, "but I recommend playing it safe and skipping it altogether if you're drinking."

Ride Smarter

With the news that extensive bike riding may lead to impotence, many men have been wondering whether it's still safe to climb on the saddle. When a man rides a bike, much of his weight is supported by the soft tissue between his pelvic bones. Since this nether region contains nerves and arteries that feed the penis, any pressure that's exerted for long periods can have serious consequences.

Harin Padma Nathan, M.D., director of the Male Clinic in Santa Monica, California, treats 50 to 100 cases of bicycle-related impotency annually, but most of them stem from falls onto the top tube. He believes that saddle compression alone probably doesn't cause the problem.

Rather, it's just one of the many factors in an aging man that can combine to sap potency. "To be diabetic, to smoke cigarettes, to have high blood pressure or cholesterol all put you at definite risk of erectile dysfunction," he explains. "But to ride a bicycle? Perhaps it's a risk. It may just aggravate other factors."

At this point, the evidence isn't compelling enough for you to hang up your wheels for good. Just be careful. If you enjoy bicycling and want to continue to ride, follow these "home remedies" for safer cycling.

Level your saddle. Or point the nose a few degrees downward to ease the pressure on your crotch.

Lower your seat. Your knees should be slightly bent when your feet are at the bottom of each pedal stroke. This allows your legs to support more of your weight.

Be wary of aero bars. These are the handlebar extensions that triathletes use. They encourage riding on the nose of the saddle, which increases crotch pressure.

Try different saddles. Find a wide style that supports your body weight on your sit bones.

Stand up and pedal every 10 minutes. This will encourage blood flow.

Use your legs as shock absorbers. Level the pedals and rise out of the saddle when riding over bumps.

Check your bike size. On a mountain bike, the top tube should be three to four inches below your crotch when you're standing over it in stocking feet. On a road bike, the clearance should be one to two inches.

Don't ignore numbness. If you experience genital numbness while riding, it's a sure sign that you're pinching the nerves and arteries.

Consider a recumbent. A recumbent bicycle can give you all the speed and thrills of an upright bike, without putting pressure on your arteries.

Index

after menopause, 248–49
oral, risks of, 233
prescription estrogens vs. herbs, 252
for protecting
 bones, 230–31, 248–49
 heart, 231–34
risks of, 232–33, 233
for treating
 endometriosis, 243
 hot flashes, 230
 vaginal dryness, 228–30
types of, 227–34
uterine fibroids, and, 235
vitamin E supplements as alternative to, 256
Eucalyptus, use in aromatherapy, 206
Eustachian tube dysfunction, 270–71
Evening primrose, for pain, 204–5
Excedrin, 196
Exercise. See also Exercises
breast cancer and, 244–45
as cause of neck pain, 270
chronic fatigue syndrome and, 170
for colds prevention, 58–59
diet and exercise program (Isaacs), 91–97
heart disease and, 276
hunger and, 127
incontinence during, 249
for job-stressed working women, 246
jumping rope, for stress relief, 76
knee pain and, 202
mind-body connection and, 152
motivational tips, 98–99
muscle mass and, 55
osteoarthritis and, 202
osteoporosis and, 55
personality and workout style, 117–25
psychological barriers to, 122–23, 124
skipping, effect on mood, 175
for sound sleep, 175–76
strength training, 8, 112–16, 169 (see also Exercises)
for stress management, 76–77
walking, 10, 53, 58–59, 77
Exercises
abdominal, 135–36
back, 133–34, 214–15
bustline/chest, 140–41
buttocks, 142–43
hip, 136–38
leg, 138–39
for stimulating mind, 149–53
for strengthening weak knees, 269
Eye problems. See Cataracts; Macular degeneration

F

Family history as heart disease risk factor, 223
Fasting plasma glucose test (FPG), 6
Fat, body, 127–28
Fatigue, preventing, with
ginseng, during menopause, 255
proper sleeping position, 173–74
water intake, 16
Fenfluramine (Rx), 126, 128
Fen-phen (Rx). See Fenfluramine (Rx)
Feverfew, migraines and, 38, 207, 278
Fiber, dietary
beans, amounts in, 11
diverticulitis and, 269
foods rich in, 32
weight loss and, 131–32
Fibersol, 131
Fibroids, uterine, 235–38
symptoms and diagnosis of, 235
treating, with alternatives to hysterectomy, 235–38
Fioricet (Rx), 197
Fiorinal (Rx), 197
First-aid, for paper cuts, 210–11
Fish
Alzheimer's disease and, 171
health benefits of, 13–14, 28
rheumatoid arthritis and, 172
as weight-loss food, 92
Fish oil, 13–14, 172
Five-minute healthy meals, 101
Flavonoids, in grape juice, 33
Flaxseed oil, for irritable bowel syndrome, 44
Fluoride, for sensitive teeth, 208–9
Folate. See Folic acid
Folic acid
heart disease and, 276
homocysteine levels and, 51, 55
sources of
 broccoli, 29
 kidney beans, 11
 oranges, 13
Foods, 9–19. See also Diet
antioxidant-rich, 30, 31, 35
fiber-rich, 32–33
five-minute healthy meals, 101
health benefits of
 apples, 30–31, 200–201
 broccoli, 9–10
 broccoli sprouts, 28–29
 cranberry juice, 287
 garlic, 10
 glutathione-rich, 31–32